Praise for
Yoga Life

"Sage and simple, playful and real, *Yoga Life* gives us permission to source our practice from within while respecting the traditions that offer us such deep peace."

—Elena Brower, bestselling author of *Practice You,*
Being You and *Softening Time*

"Bringing ancient wisdom to the modern world, *Yoga Life* is full of tools that will get you closer to your highest self with alignment, ease, and clarity."

—Sahara Rose, bestselling author and host of the
Highest Self Podcast

"With clarity and conviction, Larkin translates the medicinal magic of ancient yoga for those who need it most."

—James Nestor, *New York Times* bestselling author of
Breath: The New Science of a Lost Art

"Brett has an amazing way of making yoga accessible. This book helps you find a practice that fits the moment you're in—physically, mentally, and emotionally—in a way that's doable, even for very busy people."

—Kris Carr, *New York Times* bestselling author,
wellness activist, and cancer thriver

"Make no mistake, what is hidden behind the pages of this incredibly well-written and practical guide to yoga is the deeper meaning of the word itself: Unity. Brett Larkin acts as a powerful translator of one of the world's greatest secrets—the universal, human journey from asleep to awake."

—Katie Silcox, *New York Times* bestselling author of
Glow-Worthy and founder of the Shakti School

"From one of today's great teachers, this down-to-earth book demystifies yoga by simplifying its basic principles, and helping you find the practice that's right for you. Great for the busy Mom, the stressed-out executive, the timid-but-yoga-curious, and even the more serious practitioner who wants a break from the esoteric but still retain yoga's profound essence."

—Anodea Judith, PhD, author of *Wheels of Life*,
Eastern Body-Western Mind, and *Chakra Yoga*

"Discover the incredible impact of practicing yoga at home—a true game-changer! *Yoga Life* is your go-to book, thoughtfully crafted to accompany you on the mat. Under Brett Larkin's expert tutelage, you hold the key to enhancing your life in extraordinary ways."

—Cait Stillman, founder of ClubThrive Global

"If you're going on a yoga journey, it'd be difficult to find a better, more practical guide than *Yoga Life*: a step-by-step manual that leads us on the yogic path towards bliss, contentment, and inner wisdom."

—Dr. Chelsea Jackson Roberts, internationally celebrated yoga teacher and founder of the Yoga, Literature, and Art Camp at Spelman College Museum of Fine Art

YOGA LIFE

HABITS, POSES, AND BREATHWORK TO CHANNEL JOY AMIDST THE CHAOS

Brett Larkin

balance

NEW YORK   BOSTON

Balance
Hachette Book Group
1290 Avenue of the Americas
New York, NY 10104
GCP-Balance.com
Twitter.com/GCPBalance
Instagram.com/GCPBalance

First Edition: December 2023

Balance is an imprint of Grand Central Publishing. The Balance name and logo are trademarks of Hachette Book Group, Inc.

The publisher is not responsible for websites (or their content) that are not owned by the publisher.

The Hachette Speakers Bureau provides a wide range of authors for speaking events. To find out more, go to hachettespeakersbureau.com or email HachetteSpeakers@hbgusa.com.

Balance books may be purchased in bulk for business, educational, or promotional use. For information, please contact your local bookseller or the Hachette Book Group Special Markets Department at special.markets@hbgusa.com.

Original illustrations by Kati Lacker

Library of Congress Cataloging-in-Publication Data has been applied for.

ISBNs: 978-1-5387-2609-9 (trade paperback); 978-1-5387-2610-5 (ebook)

Printed in the United States of America

LSC-C

Printing 1, 2023

Contents

Introduction

There's a New Kind of Yoga in Town

I knew I had hit rock bottom when I was sitting at the dinner table, seventeen tabs open on my laptop, simultaneously feeding my infant and wishing my dad were dead. I was the sole caregiver for my father during his life-ending battle with cancer. At the same time, I was a first-time mom caring for my newborn son, managing the explosive growth of my business, and unpacking boxes from our move to a state where I knew no one and had no support network. All I could feel was shame. I had wanted the business success. I had wanted to start a family and to move. I had wanted my beloved father to live with me for what turned out to be the last year of his life. So I had taken on the Herculean task of moving him across the country, out of full-time nursing care, and into my apartment. But now it was too much. I felt like I was drowning. I wanted it all to be over.

Worse still, I felt like a fraud. Here I was, an award-winning yoga instructor with hundreds of thousands of followers, teaching people from all over the world about the importance of a daily morning practice through my YouTube channel and Uplifted Yoga training programs, cheerleading for them to make it happen. Meanwhile, in the chaos of my "new normal" I could barely get to the mat most days, let alone show up to my favorite sixty-minute studio class.

I was trying my best to make it all work. But I couldn't change my father's illness. I couldn't change how much my newborn demanded of me. I couldn't change how much my employees relied on me. I couldn't change my craving for calm and sanity. I was at my breaking point, and something *had* to change. Then, one horrific night while sobs and suffering echoed from every room of my apartment, I had an epiphany: What had to change wasn't my commitment to yoga; it was the yoga *itself*. I needed a new kind of practice that could keep me afloat when I was drowning. There had to be a way that yoga's brilliant wisdom, which had grounded me all these years, could still fit into my complicated and messy life of diapers and bedpans.

YOGA OF AWARENESS

When I talk about using yoga as a vehicle for personal development, most of my students think: *Ashram! White light pouring down over your head! Ethereal sounds wafting through a dim candlelit room!* I too used to buy into the belief that yoga was profound or meaningful only if it looked like a scene from *Eat Pray Love*; that it required a global tour of three continents, a monastery, a cave, silence, and a luxury eco-retreat where rich white women in skintight leggings pretzel themselves into Insta-worthy poses. And when we're not focusing on the aesthetics, we're focusing on the physicality—pushing ourselves to complete a "good workout," get a deep stretch, or achieve increasingly complex poses. All this has been overemphasized, taken out of context, and misunderstood as yoga has exploded throughout the West.

What I've come to realize in the years since my rock-bottom despair is that yoga goes *far* beyond poses. Harnessing the ancient power of yoga—the breathwork, the meditation, and the ability to adapt the postures to your unique body's needs—empowers you not only to slay your real-world problems but also to align with your most joyful self. Even if the circumstances that surround you are less than ideal. Yoga isn't about a *reprieve* from daily life, a sixty-minute Band-Aid temporarily transporting you *away* from your problems. It's an ancient science designed to help you *solve* your problems and *infuse* brilliance into whatever chaos you're facing. When practiced in its original spirit, yoga isn't about escape—it draws you more deeply into the reality of your life. You feel more deeply. Love more wholeheartedly. Enjoy an authentic intimacy with yourself and others that revitalizes your perspective.

I've realized yoga was always meant to be practiced in a way that's profoundly personal, deliciously adaptable, and above all practical. At its best, your authentic yoga has the power to widen the lens of your awareness and give you more breadth, depth, and creativity in solving whatever challenge looms in front of you right now. Uncovering the right yogic techniques for your unique mind-body-spirit constitution places you firmly on the throne of your life, nourished, reinvigorated, and joy filled. Your yoga, your way, empowers you to walk through life with an elevated and grace-filled perspective. And it's always accessible. Not as a physical pose, but as a mindset, one that's only a few breaths away.

This yoga—what I call Yoga of Awareness—is the yoga that allowed me to reclaim my sanity and create a practice that brings me closer to my best possible self as a wife, CEO, daughter, and mom, even during extreme challenges. And good news: You don't need to master fancy postures or conquer Sanskrit to improve your life using this personalized yoga. All you need is an open mind and a willingness to try ancient tools proven to make you happier, healthier, calmer, more creative, and more connected to your joy-filled essence.

A LITTLE BIT ABOUT ME

Yoga is my life's purpose, literally. I'm the founder of an award-winning yoga YouTube channel with more than half a million subscribers. Through my company, Uplifted Yoga, I've certified over four thousand yoga teachers, and through my online programs, I've helped thousands harness the healing power of yoga to fuel a personal change. After quitting my corporate job to dedicate my life to yoga, I was one of the first teachers to move all my yoga content online in 2015 (five years before the COVID-19 pandemic), and I credit the Yoga of Awareness for this foresight. I actually credit the Yoga of Awareness for *all* my success: my business, my rock-star student base and team, my soulmate husband, my beautiful sons, and my dream home.

The only way I achieved this success was through intense experimentation and adapting overlooked yogic tools like breathwork and meditation to match the challenging real-life moment I found myself in. I became determined to solve any problem I faced—from heavy traffic to existential crisis—with yoga. I dug into the history books and got back to yoga's ancient roots. I personalized everything and rediscovered what yoga *actually* is, using ancient texts as my guide. What I found became the basis of the Uplifted Yoga approach and the three foundational beliefs of my practice...

1. **Mix and Match:** The yoga style (like hatha, vinyasa, or yin) you choose is not the problem, nor is it a solution. You can't renovate a house using just a hammer, and the same goes for your personal transformation. In order to overcome your undesired habits, integrate your wide-ranging emotions, and solve your day-to-day problems, you need an adaptable yoga tool kit—one that pulls from many styles, poses, habits, and

techniques. Since they all have value, this breadth and variety is what helps you transform and balance your energy...and come into alignment with your truest, most vibrant self.

2. **Personalize:** We are all unique and ever-changing. So the idea of one-size-fits-all yoga is absurd. In order for your yoga to potently expand your awareness and improve your daily life, you need to prioritize the practices and poses that serve to balance YOU. The combination of postures, breathwork, and meditations that works well for one person may not work well for you at all—and that's a good thing! Let's uncover the magic combination of yogic techniques that fuels your emotional, physical, and spiritual evolution. So that you become the most authentic, joyful version of YOU.

3. **Adapt:** Many yoga devotees excel when attending long-form in-person group classes. But place them in a hotel room, in an airport, or on a cold floor with no mat and only ten minutes of kid-free time? They probably have no idea what to practice, or they don't do any yoga at all. Nobody teaches the skill of yogic adaptability, but I think it's the definition of advanced practice. Being "good" at yoga isn't about achieving "perfect" poses. It's about fitting in an imperfect practice that serves to nourish you in the imperfect moment you're in. Even one moment of breathwork in the midst of chaos is worthwhile. With the right set of personalized tools, you'll always know how to coax yourself back into balance. Better still, you'll begin to crave your practice instead of feeling as if it's another to-do.

Mastering this skill of *yogic adaptability*, the self-awareness to adapt your practice to the moment you're in—physically, mentally, emotionally, and spiritually—changes how you move through life.

We'll do this together by exploring a variety of yogic tools. We'll experiment to see which combination of breathwork, poses, and meditation lights YOU up inside. And we'll embrace this key paradigm shift: Instead of thinking of yoga as this "thing you do" or "place you go," imagine your whole life is a yoga studio. You're going to insert the brilliance of this ancient technology into your jam-packed day, even if it's just here and there between other activities.

WHY THIS BOOK IS DIFFERENT

Most yoga books will tell you to practice physical postures on a mat and prescribe you a specific yoga "style" with rules to follow. These books tend to assume you are already flexible and fit, with a closet full of fancy yoga pants. Instead, I'm going to assume your life is complicated, your laundry hamper is full, and time constraints or physical limitations prevent you from practicing many—or *any*—physical yoga poses. This is not a problem. I'll provide guidance so you can transform your life through the Yoga of Awareness, even if you never make it to a mat. Whether you're a proud *yogini* princess, a couch potato with an aversion to lululemon, or someone in between, you will benefit from this book.

You don't have to do complicated physical postures to receive yoga's profound benefits. What you need is your *own* unique style and way of moving. If you've felt excluded from yoga before, let me welcome you—my yoga is rooted in radical acceptance and inclusivity. I'm going to show you that everything—how, when, where, and even *what* you practice—is adaptable. Your body size, fitness, flexibility, anxiety level, gender, race, and religious background should never prevent you from feeling these tools are accessible to you. This book is about creating a safe, welcoming place on and off the mat, especially for women, people of color, curvy humans, inflexible people, folks with disabilities, the LGBTQ+ community, survivors of abuse, pre- and postnatal humans, open minds, and beautiful bodies of all shapes and sizes. I'm so grateful to my incredible and diverse Uplifted community of students and yoga teacher training graduates from across the globe who shared their stories for this book.

It's time to practice yoga in a way that embraces exactly who you are, in all your beautiful uniqueness. Yoga is about action, not aesthetics. Elevated awareness, not expensive athleisure wear. It's about evolving your life, not just sculpting your butt.

Yoga doesn't have to be complicated for you to reap the benefits. So let's get a few things straight:

- Twenty minutes is enough, as long as you pick techniques that meet your current needs.
- You don't need to be ultraflexible or able to do a headstand.
- Your practice should adapt to *you*, not the other way around— you are in the driver's seat. Shorten, lengthen, or change it completely in order to support what's going on in your life.
- You don't need to master a lot of poses—six to eight will do the trick.
- Yoga doesn't just happen on the mat. You can practice anywhere, anytime.
- You don't need to wear yoga pants. Yoga is for everyone—all bodies, all abilities, full stop.

In this book I'll share with you the decision-making framework I developed to design my own twenty-minute personalized yoga practice, which has been enhanced and refined through my work with thousands of students. Together we'll discover an adaptable yoga that can pull you out of your darkest moments and uncover your best self. A practice you can stay consistent with, even when life is throwing you a curveball. Your yoga should remind you that joy is your birthright and heal the most important relationship in your life, the one with *yourself*.

YOUR MOST IMPORTANT RELATIONSHIP

I've found that students turn to my online classes because they feel overwhelmed by life. Through emails, comments, and DMs, my students tell me they're weighed down by their emotions—they're angry, resentful, and exhausted. Many confide they're stuck in patterns of self-sabotage. Or that they feel like victims of other people or external circumstances. This manifests in anxiety, career or marital dissatisfaction, stress, high blood pressure, insomnia, binge eating, infertility, or autoimmune problems. They want to rediscover their intuition. Reclaim their inner voice. But they have been so focused on a seemingly endless list of *external* problems that they don't know how to turn *inward*.

According to yoga, all the relationships in your life are a mirror—an invitation to return to the most important and enduring relationship—the one with *you*. You know that best friend who always picks up the phone and will talk you through your breakdown while you're sobbing and stuffing your face with chocolate-covered pretzels? The bosom buddy who'll talk you off the ledge, comfort and heal you? There's a friend like that who *lives inside you*, and yoga helps you meet her.

Yoga teaches you *how* to be that BFF for yourself. Sometimes it may mean trusting this friend deep inside, even though what she's asking you to do seems *insanely* bold, contrarian, or ambitious. Yoga helps you strengthen your faith in your inner voice. It deepens the sacred relationship within so you can show up for all your other relationships calm and serene.

WHERE ARE YOU—RIGHT NOW?

I've told you about me, now I'm curious about you. The Yoga of Awareness is about meeting yourself where you are, in the moment of now, so let's check in. How are you feeling? (It's OK to be a combo.)

You're Skeptical...

You may have tried yoga in the past...by doing whatever YouTube video popped up in your phone search (hopefully one of mine!) or by going to whatever studio is closest to your house with whatever random teacher was teaching at that time.

You may think yoga won't work for you because the one time you tried it, the teacher went too fast, or the pose you tried hurt your knee, or you felt like an inflexible klutz in the back row.

Modern yoga doesn't just feel intimidating—it *is* intimidating. Why? Because it's depicted by thin beautiful women in expensive designer spandex (or sometimes thong bikinis) doing acrobatics, occasionally in pairs. Exhausting, right? I get it. After more than fifteen years of daily yoga, I still can't lift my leg into a perfect ninety-degree standing split. These types of images intimidate me too, and I'm an award-winning teacher. This far-from-realistic portrayal of yoga may have made you feel inadequate, or maybe it made you feel you had to be sexy, or more spiritual, more vegan, more into essential oils and sage, and never use a plastic straw in order to fit in. The bottom line: These disempowering images of yoga promote the idea *not to be YOU*!

My Promise: You don't need to set foot on a mat to take advantage of what I share in this book. The poses I present are streamlined, based on what I've seen works best for a diverse student population and the unique souls and bodies of my over four thousand teaching graduates. On a tough day, you can practice what I call "Yoga

Habits," even from the safety of your couch. I urge you to adopt a set of yogic tools you love and indulge in them as you please. The best part? There's no need to be perfect. Let's celebrate you as you are in this moment. You're already enough.

You're Too Busy...

You've mastered certain yoga poses and have a home practice, but you crave a deeper transformation. You picked up this book because you're curious about how yoga can fuel your personal development to improve your life and relationships. But you can't imagine fitting one more thing into your day.

My Promise: Everything I present is about deepening your practice and generating practical results in *less* time, not more. With an active toddler, a new baby, and my demanding business running a team of twelve to help thousands of wonderful students, my life is jam-packed. I often feel the same way you do. With so many demands on my time, it can feel as if there's nothing left for ME. The techniques in my yoga tool kit save me daily, even when I'm on the go and nowhere near a mat. I will never ask you to carve out hours each day. Twenty minutes a day is more than enough. If these yoga tools work for my time-crunched life, they'll work for yours too.

You're Recovering from an Injury or a Health Issue...

Perhaps weight lifting, running, or even vigorous yoga caused injury to your body. Or maybe physical limitations make it challenging to find yoga that feels doable for you. You'd love to experience yoga's healing benefits, but it's been hard to find a style that fits your body's needs.

My Promise: I will not leave you behind. Everything in this book is about you meeting *your* soulmate postures. Personalization and adaptability are the focus of this book. You'll reach the end with a unique, tailor-made practice that works for YOU and YOUR BODY, exactly as it is in this moment.

You're All In...

You're a yoga devotee and eager to start personalizing your own sequences. Maybe you're a yoga teacher. But you're inhibited by the "yoga police," fearful of trying things that are different from what you've been taught. You're ready to go behind the scenes and break down the how and why of yoga class design. You want to take yogic philosophy out of books and into your daily problem-solving. Or take your meditation and breathwork to the next level. You want to harness the potential of these practices to improve your energy, mood, and creativity—to propel your transformation.

My Promise: This book will give you the confidence you need to accelerate into your personal next level—and become your own best teacher. As you explore and adapt your practice to suit yourself and your own needs, your relationships and life off the mat will be uplifted.

HOW TO USE THIS BOOK

I designed our yoga road trip in two main parts, with a bonus guide for exceptional circumstances, like pregnancy or injury. You'll get the most out of this book if you move through the chapters in order.

Part I breaks down the basics of my Yoga of Awareness philosophy, clearing up confusing yoga myths, styles, and misunderstood terms. You'll discover your mind-body constitution (what yogis call a *dosha*). You'll embrace the poses and yoga styles that best suit YOUR needs (and avoid the ones that undermine you). To experience extra yoga sparkle in your day, I'll help you set up your home practice space and show you ways to channel your happiest self—without ever touching a mat.

In part II we'll design your very own personalized yoga tool kit, walking step-by-step through the five elements—breath, warm-up, movement, stretching, and meditation—that sync to your mood, energy level, and goals. You can perform these practices in the order I provide for a cohesive yoga ritual or mix and match techniques depending on what challenges you're facing at the moment. This is where you'll meet the soulmate yoga postures that will drastically improve your life and connect you to your most joyful self. Each chapter includes a quiz that matches you to the ideal postures and practices for your personality. And, as always, if you can't make it to the mat (or don't want to!), we'll be talking about off-the-mat Yoga Habits so you can leverage this ancient wisdom without getting physical.

Finally, at the back of the book (page 241), you'll find an adaptations guide for beginners, easing anxiety, pregnancy, your period, menopause, losing weight, and recovering from an injury, all customized for your unique energy type. If you hit a major bump in the road in life, this appendix provides tips, resources, and templates so you can further personalize your practice or aid your students.

All three sections are designed to support you in aligning with your most authentic, joy-filled life. And yes, I include tools and techniques for the "crazy days" when you may not make it to your yoga mat.

YOGA CAN HANDLE ALL OF YOU

Before we officially begin, I want to share with you a moment from smack in the middle of my rock bottom. That thought about my dying father that brought me so much shame? How I was feeling so overwhelmed that I wished he would just die already so I'd have one fewer thing to take care of? Well, ten days later, he did.

My dad had a few hours of remarkable mental clarity five days before he died. It was as if a veil lifted around his hospital-style bed in my guest room. Miraculously, my disoriented cancer patient was gone and my dad was back!

While he had this window of lucidity, I helped him make calls to those he loved most. He cracked jokes with his beloved cousins and sister. He called friends. While I lingered outside the door, he even had a beautiful conversation with my mom, who had divorced him thirty years before. I stayed close to his side, relishing these moments when he was his old self. That same afternoon, I sensed this window of clarity closing. Once again the fatigue started to take over, and his personality slipped away. Dad returned to his former state, that of a semiconscious cancer patient. His breathing became more labored. All medical signs showed he was in a steep decline. I cleared my schedule, paid someone to babysit, and just sat next to his bed. I thought he was asleep when suddenly he murmured, "You always surprise me."

I felt confused. "Dad, what do you mean? How?"

"By how good you are," he said, truly *looking* at me with an exhausted smile. I knew at that moment that my dad wasn't just referring to what a good caretaker I'd tried to be (despite feeling like a failure most of the time). He was talking about me as a person. In that moment he saw beyond every flaw, into my core. He was saying that it had filled him up to see my goodness grow and ripen throughout both our lives.

I think about this phrase a lot when it comes to my relationship with yoga. I often find myself on my mat, dazed after a practice, thinking: *You always surprise me, yoga. By how good you are.*

I come to yoga with whatever I'm feeling. Whether it's hurt, rage, disappointment, fear, or petty annoyance, yoga never ceases to surprise me with the magical way it transforms me from the inside out. How it lightens my pain and problems. How it makes me feel better, brighter, more purposeful.

In this book, you will find a tool kit of practices, both physical exercises and lifestyle habits, so yoga can become the reliable best friend you always wanted—but didn't know you needed. It's definitely *not* about touching your toes or becoming religious. It's about practical ways to improve your life. The calm and clarity you're seeking are available to you now—you just need the right tool at the right moment. These ancient tools of yoga just might surprise you, by how good they are.

Part I

Yoga Habits for a Happier You

CHAPTER 1

Yoga Is Awareness

Conquer the Negative Voices in Your Head

Looking at my life as an online yoga mogul—over half a million YouTube subscribers, running international certification programs with thousands of students—you'd probably think a career in yoga had always been my plan, right? Nothing could be further from the truth. During my online yoga trainings, students often ask what brought me to yoga. When did I realize this form of exercise was "the one"? Well, as many great loves do, it started with a crush.

ORIGIN STORY: LIFE BEFORE YOGA

My motive for trying yoga had nothing to do with wellness, health, an injury, or personal betterment. In college I harbored a crush on this hippie Croatian classmate and was desperate for him to notice me. At the time he was really into meditation, and I was letting go of my high-school dream of becoming a professional dancer. Always a competitive movement junkie, I'd switched to practicing hard-core Pilates, but my cute Croatian, with his adorable accent, kept suggesting I take up yoga.

"But...," I'd respond, confused. "Why? Yoga is for wimps."

In a last-ditch effort to get out of the friend zone, I decided to try yoga, but only if it was the *most* intense kind. I found Bikram Yoga (athletic, hard-core yoga that takes place in a heated room) and, both surprisingly and not...an addiction developed.

Flashforward six weeks: I'm staring in the mirror at a spandex-clad woman in the front row, trying to out-yoga her. She was best in class at the 6:00 p.m. sweat-fest in SoHo—always in the coveted front-row-center spot wearing an awe-inspiring, barely-there black outfit. I'd compete with her in the mirror from the second row, trying to hold each pose longer than she. Yes: I'd found a way to make even yoga a competition. I craved more. I wanted to be *the best*.

All that competition worked my body so hard that it started to burn off a layer of tension and anxiety I hadn't even known I lived with. After boiling myself in insanely hot yoga for weeks, I calmed down enough to get curious. Could it make sense to explore forms of yoga that didn't end with me in the center of a puddle of sweat? I cautiously decided to venture beyond Bikram. Turning to the early-2000s internet, I found a simple online hatha yoga routine with now-famous teacher Jason Crandell. In my (charmingly?) compulsive way, I followed along with that same twenty-minute video every. Single. Day. My yoga addiction really kicked into gear when I stepped away from the studio (and away from any potential nemesis in the studio mirror). Practicing in my apartment, in my own space, made me feel more powerful in my own life.

In less than three months, I started to see the results of my dedication: I was less anxious, and my brain's never-ending loop of self-judgment seemed fainter. I even found myself becoming less competitive and more focused on...me? Goodbye, Croatian boy—I had found real love! Yoga became a security blanket that I couldn't live without. I clung to my yoga mat—even taking it on a spring break girls' trip to Miami, where my friends rolled their eyes when I told them I had to practice. I had zero knowledge of yogic alignment or philosophy. I didn't even know what I was accessing. I just knew I was less stressed and calmer. Once I felt I knew enough not to make a total fool of myself in Downward Dog and Warrior 2 Pose, I decided to seek out a human teacher in an unheated room. I hit the streets of New York to speed-date some yoga studios that weren't the sticky-hot Bikram type.

FALLING IN YOGA LOVE

It's apt in many ways that my journey into yoga was romantically motivated, since yoga became one of the most passionate romances of my life. My love affair with the Croatian cutie never panned out, but what was supposed to be a dalliance with yoga went from an intense fling to steady and serious when I found my studio and people at ISHTA Yoga in Manhattan. Alan Finger and his team of teachers created the ideal learning environment for me to recover from my anxiety-fueled hypercompetitiveness and reinvent myself.

Up to this point, my life had been primarily about winning—the date, the job, the glamorous life—and avoiding disaster, which I told myself was lurking right around the corner. I was constantly strategizing ways to become *perfect*. I thought six steps ahead to avoid anything going wrong. My anxiety levels were through the roof, since trying to optimize every second of my life was *exhausting*. To top it all off, I was immensely hard on myself. If there were an Academy Award for negative self-talk and worst-case-scenario predictions, I'd have statues lining my mantel. I was walking through life pressurized and mildly panic-stricken. And I would still be to this day, if it hadn't been for *one moment* that changed everything.

It's Thursday-evening yoga class, and I'm shoehorning myself into the deepest possible Pigeon Pose (a floor stretch that shock waves my knee and hip with pain). My teacher's gentle voice said, "Notice if you've gone too far in this pose." She paused and walked my way. Her next words seared deep into my brain: "If you've pushed yourself too far in this stretch, to the point of discomfort, it's likely you push yourself too hard in life too."

BOOM.

Somewhere in my terrified, control-oriented mind, a light bulb came on, and I realized *I had a choice.* The choice to stop pushing myself into the deepest stretch and to practice kindness toward myself instead. Cautiously, awkwardly, I backed out of my extreme Pigeon into a sensation that felt more easeful. Then I exploded into tears.

That Thursday night, the icy tyrant inside me—the voice that wanted to control every outcome, win every point, avoid catastrophe, do everything *perfectly*—started to melt.

Something about this kindly yoga teacher's voice, her compassionate comment in that precise moment, showed me that the crack-the-whip, cruel voice in my head wasn't *me*. That perhaps I didn't *have* to listen to it. There had been a tyrannical program running in my brain for over a decade like malware, telling me to strive, to achieve, no matter the consequences. But it didn't have to be that way.

I finally saw the difference between thinking from my default programming and thinking from a new, curious, compassionate space. My default programming came from a place of no awareness in which my panicked inner strategist reigned as usual. The new thoughts came from a place of elevated awareness, with my highest self questioning everything my inner strategist assumed was true. You, like me, were programmed by society and your family. Without awareness, these inherited, unconscious, physical-emotional programs run the show of your life into your adulthood, like bad habits you can't see. The good news? You have the power to change the script. Take a look...

Default Program (No Awareness): *Push harder, stretch deeper, be the best!*

New Thought (Yoga of Awareness): *Why am I so mean to myself? I don't need to push so hard. I'm telling myself a story that if I'm not the best, I'm not worthy of love. What if that's not true?*

Over time, while stretching in yoga or practicing meditation, I got to know a slew of other villains living rent-free in my head. Negative Nancy, Debbie Downer, Cruella de Vil, and *all* their frenemies, vying for my brain's attention. As I deepened my breath, instead of innocently believing them, I could relax and think: *I have a choice. I don't have to listen to any of you.* The more I practiced, the more I realized the voices in my head weren't the real me.

If you think this sounds "woo-woo," I don't blame you. But science backs this up. Here's how it works: Say you choose to tell yourself, *I'm the worst person ever.* Over time, a voice in your head reinforces that thought—that what you're telling yourself is true. The idea becomes a groove in your brain. Author, academic, and social psychologist Brené Brown calls this "story making."[1] Your brain wants to reinforce whatever reality you choose to tell yourself. It encodes the stories you tell yourself into your neural pathways for easy access. In the words of neuroscientist Donald Hebb, "Neurons that fire together, wire together."[2]

The good news? Yoga grants you the power to rewire your brain by synchronizing your breath and body. This slows your thoughts down, coaxing them to rearrange themselves in ways outside of their usual groove. New neural pathways form, creating kinder, more empowering voices in your head.

Talent agents have the challenge of managing divas (of all gender identities!) who are often irrational. As a human, you have the challenge of managing the unwieldy peanut gallery of characters in your head (like Statler and Waldorf on *The Muppet Show*). Some spiritual lineages refer to these voices in your head as "the ego." But I like to think of them as a cast of characters who tell you stories all day. The more you tap into the Yoga of Awareness, the more you see that the drama they're putting on isn't necessarily true.

> Brené Brown advises watching your thoughts by saying: "*The story I'm telling myself about this is _____.*"

What you put in that blank is often negatively skewed, hypothetical, or maybe not even factually accurate. In my Pigeon Pose, the story I was telling myself was, *The teacher will judge me if I don't go into my deepest stretch. If I'm not feeling some pain, I'm probably not doing the stretch right. I should try harder. I should be better.*

For some people, simply asking, *What is the story I'm telling myself?* is enough to gain perspective and evolve their inner dialogue. For me, I couldn't get my nervous system regulated enough to even ponder such a question without practicing yoga and meditation first. After years of negative predictions, cruel self-talk, and wiring my body and brain to high alert, my nervous system was in a near-constant state of alarm. I needed yoga as a first step, before I could even *think* clearly.

See, by soothing your central nervous system, yoga can get you out of fight-or-flight mode and bring your thinking brain back online. Yogis understand that your body and brain are in a reciprocal relationship. If you slow down your breath, you slow down your thoughts. The more space between your thoughts, the more awareness you gain of the voices in your head. It's the body and mind working together, reinforcing one another to relax and slow down, that makes yoga extra powerful.

Yoga empowers you to choose which voices in your head you tune in to, and which you tune out. At first I could tap into the Yoga of

Awareness only during or immediately after a physical yoga class. But within a few weeks, I found I could tap into the Yoga of Awareness in all sorts of situations...at any time.

I could change the story—about myself...At home...

Default Program (No Awareness): *I have to stay up late to vacuum and unload the dishwasher—and I'm so tired. Life is so unfair.*

New Thought (Yoga of Awareness): *I have a story that I'm not worthy of love if my kitchen doesn't look perfect.*

At the office...

Default Program (No Awareness): *I should outsource this complicated project, but I'd rather just do it myself so I know it's done right.*

New Thought (Yoga of Awareness): *I have a story about the quality of others' work that blocks me from receiving help and prevents me from having better work-life balance.*

Socially...

Default Program (No Awareness): *I have to go to this event, even though there are a million other ways I'd rather spend my time. This sucks.*

New Thought (Yoga of Awareness): *I have a story that if I decline this invitation, I'll be unsafe or unloved in some way. What's stopping me from politely declining and creating some healthy boundaries so my life feels fun?*

If you're wondering where your default programs come from... look at your family. You didn't just inherit your mother's nose and your father's eyebrows. You inherited their survival programs—their fears, their beliefs about success and safety, the legacies of their traumas—which have likely been passed down through generations.[3] Unless you work to change them, these live on in *your* mind.

The voices inside your head may come from your posse of friends too—aka peer pressure. These chattering minions have overrun the stage instead of making way for the real star in this performance of your life—the authentic *you*.

Some of this subconscious familial and societal programming can be helpful. For example, my father reinforced principles in my formative years that turned me into an entrepreneur. (Thank you, Dad!) But much of what we internalize from our caregivers is fear-based and unhelpful. The good news: Yoga gives you awareness of it all. Once you can see your programming, you can choose to keep what you love and let go of what no longer serves you. In yoga we call this evolution of our default conditioning *karma*.[4]

A Note on Sanskrit Terms

If you're new to yoga, it can seem as if there are a *lot* of new terms and ideas to master. I often see students get overwhelmed and confused by Sanskrit. If that's you, don't panic. We are going to use Sanskrit terms to honor the centuries-long tradition of yogic wisdom, but I promise they're not as complicated as they may seem on first read. Take your time, and feel free to refer to the glossary on page 269 if you need a refresher at any point.

HEALING FAST AND SLOW— THE ROLE OF KARMA

Karma may be yoga's most popular (and most wildly misunder-stood!) philosophical concept. Most people think of karma as the club where Snooki became famous on *Jersey Shore* or this scary mechanism the universe uses to dish out well-deserved punish-ments. But that's not what it is at all. *Karma* is a Sanskrit word that means "action" or "deed." These are the lessons we learn throughout our lives that challenge us to grow.

> **Karma:** The lessons you need to integrate into this lifetime to discover your joy-filled authentic self.

Karma presents you with the opportunity to choose: Will you learn and grow from this challenge? Or will you stay stuck in old patterns? Think of moving through your karma as the process of softening, unwinding, and dissolving your habitual stress responses and fear-based programs.

Every person on the planet will move through their karma—the question is how you want to do it. You can move through your karma slowly, resisting the same lesson over and over. You can squirm and struggle while life continues to present your karma to you in a vari-ety of scenarios, patiently waiting for you to learn and grow. OR you can use the Yoga of Awareness to move through your karma swiftly, learning the lessons you need to learn in order to evolve gracefully and efficiently, with a smile on your face and peace in your heart.

Practicing yoga created the nervous system conditions and men-tal clarity I needed to realize *I had a choice.* That moment when I backed out of that Pigeon Pose, even though my habitual internal dialogue was coaxing me to stretch as far as I could go? That was a karmic moment. I chose something *other* than my default pattern.

> **Karmic moment:** A moment when you use the Yoga of Awareness to choose something different from your habitual patterns.

Life is full of karmic moments. Every day, you're presented with scenarios in which you can respond *unintentionally* from old programming (lesson *not* learned) or respond *intentionally* by bringing awareness to the moment, choosing a different response, and moving through life in a new way (lesson learned). It's why you may end up in the same kind of job, or dating the same kind of person, even though you switched careers and moved across the country to get away from their doppelganger. Each moment becomes a choice to stay the same or evolve into an even better version of you.

If you're not sure how to make this shift, don't worry. The rest of this book is here to help. Together we'll be designing a yoga practice to support your evolution to greater awareness. But first we need to learn an ancient framework that serves as the fuel for this kind of transformational yoga. Leveraging the age-old wisdom of Ayurveda empowers you to personalize your yoga in such a way that you move through your karma with grace.

YOGA HAS A SISTER: MEET AYURVEDA

In the West yoga has been cast as an only child. Truth? It was always meant to be understood in the context of its sister science, Ayurveda. Translated from Sanskrit, *Ayurveda* literally means "life knowledge."[5] Starting nearly three millennia ago in India, Ayurveda evolved into a galaxy of holistic and healing therapies. At its core

Ayurveda is about creating balance in the body and spirit with a focus on your individual mind-body constitution. Ayurveda's a vast interwoven system that addresses everything from nutrition to mind-body consciousness. In this book I'm zooming in on one of its most fundamental concepts: the *doshas*—the three elements believed to be present in each person's body and mind. Together, the three elements result in your personal constitution. Think of your Ayurvedic constitution as being like your zodiac sign in astrology. It enables you to personalize how you move through life.

 AIR (*Vata*): Energetic, creative, lively.

 FIRE (*Pitta*): Strong willed, determined, decisive.

EARTH (*Kapha*): Steady, stable, with high stamina.

Interestingly enough, the Sanskrit word *dosha* literally translates to "that which can cause problems."[6] Why? Well, when these elements are balanced within us, we're healthy. But when one element skews out of balance, problems crop up, either as disease or as mental patterns that keep us stuck in our karma. The catch? Balance looks different for each of us.

According to Ayurveda, each person is a mixture of all three of the elements, with one being dominant.[7] The goal is *not* to bring all your elements into equal thirds, but to find the combination of these three elements at which you're operating as your best, most authentic, most joyful self. For example, maybe your best self shines through when you're mostly grounded and stable (*kapha*), with just a dash of creativity and determination to complement (*vata* and *pitta*). It's in that winning balance that you feel your best, think most clearly, and move through your karma fastest.

What happens to most of us, however, is that without awareness, our dominant element gains momentum, snowballing as it runs the show in our minds and bodies.

Yoga was designed to help us balance these three elements, with different poses and techniques aimed at tempering or enhancing the air, fire, and earth within us. So knowing which is dominant in you is pivotal to understanding what yogic techniques you should indulge in and which ones you should avoid. Once you know your dominant element, you instantly gain more awareness of your habitual tendencies, likes, dislikes, desires, and aversions, and the common themes of the voices running amok in your head. Understanding your elemental makeup empowers you to make adjustments in all areas of your life, just as your zodiac sign is essential in astrology to understanding your horoscope. The goal is to personalize your yoga practice to soothe your dominant element and discover what balance feels like, so you can operate in the world as your happiest, highest self. Understanding your dominant *dosha* is essential to your personalized practice. So which is most dominant within you?

MEET THE *DOSHAS*

How to discern your dominant element? It's easier than you think. Let's look at the personalities that result from air (*vata*), fire (*pitta*), and earth (*kapha*) dominance respectively. Each element has different strengths as well as different negative programs that are running the show in your mind. Maybe you'll recognize yourself in one (or all!) of these personality types.

Two quick notes before we dive in: First, I've simplified these personality profiles to make the core concepts easy to understand. Please know that Ayurveda is a *highly* nuanced science. If you'd like to go into more depth, I'd recommend my dear friend Sahara Rose Ketabi's book *Ayurveda (Idiot's Guides),* or Michelle S. Fondin's *The Wheel of Healing with Ayurveda.* For now we're going to stick to the basics.

AIR (Vata)

You are a visionary or artist, bubbling with ideas. Your creativity leads you in so many exciting directions, but you get easily overwhelmed. As a child maybe you loved to draw, sing, and paint. Today you might be a freelance photographer, artist, or other creative. You're expressive and emotional and feel most alive when *creating*. You're great at starting projects but not so great at finishing them, and you are often frustrated that there's not enough time to manifest all your ideas. On the yoga mat, you love to flow and raise your energy through backbends and breathwork. You're naturally flexible and most comfortable when in movement. You have massive talent, but you do *not* like to look at your QuickBooks. You haven't organized it in months, and you can't find the sticky note where you wrote your password.

> *Vata* **Comfort Zone:** Creation. When things get too practical and boring, your interest fades. You like to think about the big picture. No one should come to you with all the nitty-gritty details of a task.
>
> *Vata* **Out of Balance:** When your air gets too high, it results in you feeling overwhelmed. You feel paralyzed by a million ideas, which results in an inability to focus or implement. You're confused, overwhelmed, irrational, dramatic, hypersensitive, perfectionistic.
>
> *Vata* **in Balance:** You discern your most promising ideas and channel them into tangible results. This is when you're a visionary: creative, aligned, fulfilled, soulful, magnetic, open to collaboration.
>
> **Default Want:** Everything? You can't decide!
>
> **Challenge:** To follow through. You need to create separate containers for the ideas that truly matter and finish them.

FIRE (*Pitta*)

As a fiery *pitta* you're an incredible team leader and the person who has an hour-by-hour itinerary, even if you're on a quick day trip to the beach. You're efficient, methodical, and organized—the consummate overachiever. On the yoga mat, just as in life, you want to win. This can result in your pushing yourself into more advanced poses (your "striving program" is strong). You're much better at doing than being, and much better at talking than listening.

> *Pitta* **Comfort Zone:** Stress. Yup. Counterintuitive as that sounds, when things get too relaxed, or "too good," you'll self-sabotage by conjuring up something that *must* be done immediately.
>
> *Pitta* **Out of Balance:** You turn from a capable captain to a bossy, fire-breathing dragon. You're irritable, impatient, judgmental, controlling.
>
> *Pitta* **in Balance:** You're a magnetic, radiant leader everyone can rely on. You're empowering, decisive, action oriented, and amazing under pressure.
>
> **Default Want:** To achieve. As a go-getting *pitta*, you're addicted to the sense of accomplishment—and ensuring admiration— that follows a hard day's work.
>
> **Challenge:** To let go of control. To simply *be* instead of do. To celebrate what you've already done and realize you are *innately* enough, without achieving more.

EARTH (*Kapha*)

As an earthy *kapha* you're the chill homebody who does *not* want to go for a run, but who *does* want to binge-watch the latest Netflix sensation. As a kid you loved knitting and collecting things like feathers and rocks. Maybe now you're a teacher, carpenter, or chef. You're grounded, levelheaded, and nurturing, and you give phenomenal advice. You tend to put others' needs before your own. Your goal is for everything to stay just the way it is now—no curveballs. When it comes to yoga, you would rather not get on the mat. Going for a walk or reading a book sounds highly preferable to getting sweaty in a yoga class.

Kapha **Comfort Zone:** Inertia. Things staying *the same*. When things get too stressful or too fast, you cope by zoning out on the couch or playing games on your phone.

Kapha **Out of Balance:** When your earth turns to heavy mud, you start procrastinating. You become tired, lethargic, depressed, unmotivated.

Kapha **in Balance:** When your earth element is in balance, you're the ultimate healer of yourself and others. You nurture others while honoring your own boundaries with a quiet confidence that uplifts everyone around you. You're reliable, steady, loving, and loyal.

Default Want: To be comfortable and avoid challenges. The less movement the better.

Challenge: To take decisive action, uphold your boundaries, and push yourself, gently, into more movement and new situations. To drag yourself out of the house, even though you'd rather spend some quality time with a book.

If you see yourself in all these characters, that's normal, because all three exist within each of us. The question is, which do you see yourself in the *most*? Check your *dosha* dominance with my miniquiz.

Quiz: Discover Your Dosha

Circle the answer that strikes you as most true the majority of the time. Don't overthink it! The *dosha* that tends to skew out of balance for you may change with the seasons, or over time, and that's perfectly OK. You can return to this quiz if you feel a shift in your energy down the road.

1. The loudest voice in my head tells me:
   a. You should be doing more! Just finish this, it's only 9:30 p.m. Sleep is for the weak!
   b. Wow, you have so many ideas and yet, what have you actually accomplished? Do you ever follow through?
   c. You can start doing this later, when life is less stressful. For now, you need to chill and lie down.
2. What energy feels the most familiar to your life?
   a. Fast paced and challenging.
   b. Flowing and spontaneous.
   c. Steady and predictable.
3. How do you make choices?
   a. I usually have a gut feeling. I weigh the pros and cons, then decide.
   b. I hate committing to just one thing. I make choices reluctantly. I usually go with how I'm feeling in any given moment.
   c. It takes me forever. I do lots of research—to the point of analysis paralysis. Sometimes I just wait to see what happens. Or I let other people decide.
4. What's your day-to-day mood?
   a. Driven, purposeful, and goal oriented.

b. Enthusiastic, excited to create.

c. Laid back and relaxed.

5. If you're under stress, how do you feel?

a. Frustrated and impatient.

b. Anxiety ridden and hypersensitive.

c. I go into isolation and withdraw.

Quiz Results + What to Do ASAP to Find Balance

If you marked more a's, your dominant element is likely fire (*pitta*). You're a natural leader. We'll talk more about how *pitta*-dominant people can use breathwork, movement, and meditation to bring a sense of calmness and pleasure to their lives. For now, here are some practical and easy off-mat actions you can take to start balancing your energy.

If You See Yourself in the Pitta Dosha

- Invite in a "cooling" element anytime you feel yourself getting stressed. When your fiery *pitta* temper flares, visualize snow, take a cold shower, or just splash your face with cold water in a pinch. Stuck in a boardroom? Visualize a waterfall overhead, cooling you down inside and out.

- Slow down! Treat yourself to an unexpected break. Engage in something fun and frivolous. Take a bath in the middle of the day. Go for a walk in the afternoon. End work a little earlier than usual and stop in at that art gallery you've been eyeing. Pause intentionally throughout the day and lie down, even for five minutes. Frequent breaks help you to respond, rather than react from that place of pure heat.

- Especially if you tend to think that the other shoe is about to drop, make it a point to enjoy the little things in life. Relish the good. Tell yourself, *It's safe for me to be happy. It's safe for me to relax.*

If you marked more b's, your dominant element is likely air (*vata*). You're an innovator and visionary. You have a million ideas (a gift!), but this can lead to confusion. Your yoga will serve to anchor your creativity in the here and now. Here are some things you can do ASAP to balance your air element.

If You See Yourself in the Vata **Dosha**

- Touch a tree or put your hands in the dirt. Every time you feel your airy *vata* energy leading you to overwhelm, get outside and put your two feet on some grass (barefoot if you can!).
- List all the ideas you have. Then just pick one. Challenge yourself to break that idea down into a series of smaller steps. Then do one baby step to make that idea become a reality.
- Commit to working on a schedule. Start writing in your journal at 8:00 a.m. sharp, and honor that pledge to yourself. *Vatas* thrive on a predictable schedule.
- Practice stillness. Resist the urge to multitask. Notice your impulse to stay in motion. Instead, stay still and breathe into your belly.
- Visualize yourself as a creative soul with a clear purpose. Tell yourself, *I trust myself. It's safe for me to focus on just this one thing. It's time to take action.*

If you marked more c's, your dominant element is likely earth (*kapha*). You'd rather enjoy a quiet dinner than a night at a dance club. You like to feel safe and comfortable and take things slow. Your yoga will serve to motivate you so you can offer your gifts to the world from a place of abundant energy. For now, experiment with these ideas to start balancing your earth energy.

If You See Yourself in the Kapha Dosha

- Force yourself to move. Take a walk around the block before you cozy up on the couch.
- Challenge yourself to do one small thing outside your comfort zone. Say hi to a stranger. Sign up for the class you've been eyeing for months. Apply for the promotion.
- Light a candle with your favorite scent at your home workspace or by the bath. Bring a little fire into your day.
- Set and uphold your boundaries. Remind yourself that it is OK to say no to other people. Put your needs first. Speak up when you'd normally stay quiet.
- Nourish yourself. Change your routine, experiment with something new in a small way. Tell yourself, *It's safe for me to make mistakes. It's safe for me to fail. It's safe to take risks.*

In the case of a close call or tie, you may have more than one element that tends to skew out of balance. There are endless *dosha* quizzes on the internet, and while they focus primarily on diet and digestion, they may offer you more insight into your full Ayurvedic constitution. Take what resonates with you and, as always, trust yourself. If you feel out of balance, it may be time to work on a different *dosha*. For example, I'm primarily fire (*pitta*) dominant, but I have high air (*vata*) as well, so I work to tame both.

ALIGNING WITH THE REAL YOU

If you were to strip away all the voices in your head, step out of your karmic patterns, and perfectly modulate your dominant *dosha*, what would that look like? What would balance of the three elemental *doshas* look like for YOU? For example, if you're fire (*pitta*) dominant, how much fire is enough? You don't want too much (exploding into flames). But you also don't want too little (shying away from your role as a guiding light to others). Next, at what levels do you want the supporting elements, air and earth, to show up so your unique style of leadership shines through?

It's time to take everything we've learned and go one layer deeper. Let's leverage the *doshas* to align with your happiest, most brilliant self.

In Ayurveda there are *two* states of being:

The Real You (*Prakriti*):[8] You in the perfect Ayurvedic ratios you were born with (let's say one-half air, one-quarter fire, one-quarter earth). Your unique balance of these elements allows the unfettered, joy-filled, balanced version of you to shine forth. This is how you were meant to be, before fears, insecurities, and all the malware crept in.

The Out-of-Balance You (*Vrakriti*):[9] This is how you're (likely) operating right now, with barnacles of negative programs and life circumstances creating a crusty layer. These legacy programs weigh you down and prevent you from embodying the authentic self you're here to reclaim. Maybe your dominant air element is too high and your fire is a little too hot. Or maybe your earth overrides everything and you feel a bit stuck.

When you're living your life out of balance (*vrakriti*), you misidentify the voices in your head as those of your true self. Awareness is the bridge that helps you move from your out-of-balance persona (*vrakriti*) and through the life lessons you need to learn (your karma), restoring you to your balanced, authentic self (*prakriti*). And yoga is what gives you this awareness. Because once you know you have a choice, you can turn down the volume on the voices and patterns that no longer serve you. You can choose to come back into alignment with your joy-filled, authentic self.

CHOOSING YOUR YOGA

A word to the wise: Don't let who you are right now (your *vrakriti*) select your yoga. In other words, don't let what you *want* stand in for what you *need*. It's a common pitfall that will result in your energy skewing even more out of balance! Think about it: Someone who is two-thirds air is likely going to be attracted to *more* air. Like attracts like. We crave what feels familiar, even if it's unhealthy for us.

Without awareness, your dominant *dosha* may lure you into yoga styles that *exacerbate* the element that's already out of balance, causing you to double down on your unhealthy tendencies. Remember how initially I focused on Bikram Yoga, competing in spandex hot pants with my black-clad nemesis in the studio mirror? Worse still for my fire element (*pitta*), Bikram is held in a hot room! *Yikes!* This was a catastrophic combination that amplified my already high fire. It felt natural to push myself like that, but it wasn't bringing me into balance.

This is one of the biggest problems with our one-size-fits-all modern yoga: the risk that it will take us *further* from our authentic selves. If you choose the wrong kind of yoga for your dominant element, you could exacerbate imbalances you already have. In Western society we already have a general imbalance with too much fire (*pitta*—"go-go-go") and too much air (*vata*—always-on work culture, social media distractions). The popular yoga styles out there today reflect this. The majority of yoga classes in our modern world increase the air and fire elements, potentially making disparities worse.

IF YOU REMEMBER ONLY ONE THING

Yoga is not just about physical poses, it's about awareness. Awareness starts with considering who you are and learning to see yourself through the lens of Ayurveda's three elements (the *doshas*). This helps you better understand yourself and the choices you tend to make. You were born as a joyful soul on this earth with a unique gift to give. When your energy is balanced, this authentic self shines through. You feel untethered, happy, and alive. Of course, growing up in our complex world, you learned (often flawed) coping mechanisms in order to survive. This default programming has resulted in a misalignment of your *doshas*, which in turn has resulted in many of the challenges you struggle with today. The Yoga of Awareness gifts you the ability to *choose*. Each time you face a *karmic* moment, will you evolve toward the real you? Or will you stay the same?

A personalized practice of breathwork, yoga poses, and meditations accelerates this evolution. We'll assemble these together in part II. But as you're about to see, yoga is even bigger than that. Because it's not exclusively on the mat that you practice this awareness; the real yoga studio is your life.

CHAPTER 2

How to Live Your Yoga

The Three Skills of Yoga in Action

"I'm so overwhelmed."

"I don't have time to practice."

"I feel isolated and unmotivated."

I hear this mixture of overwhelm and burnout from my community every day. Modern life is complex for all of us. But what if wisdom from two thousand years ago could help? We saw in chapter 1 how Ayurveda provides a lens through which we can understand our habitual tendencies and strive to balance our dominant element. But how do we put this newfound awareness into action? What guidelines do ancient yogic texts provide for living a joy-filled life?

BEYOND THE MAT: WHAT IS YOGIC WISDOM?

If you want to expand yoga's healing brilliance into your day-to-day life, yogic philosophy can help. Today we're used to seeing yoga as a physical endeavor, but until the twentieth century, it was primarily a spiritual one. Historically, in India, physical movement was only one tiny piece of yoga. Ancient yoga wasn't focused on the health of the body, but on transcending the body to achieve blissful enlightenment (*samadhi*). The body was actually seen as an obstacle to overcome. People achieved this elevated state of enlightenment through studying yogic scripture, fasting, mortifying the flesh, long periods of isolation, intense breathwork, and lots of meditation. Yogis followed a rigorous moral code that prescribed what they could and could not do—for example, engaging in sexual intercourse was forbidden. Throughout most of history, this yogic wisdom was reserved for two groups of people: young men training for priesthood and the elderly. In ancient Indus Valley civilizations, "retirement" meant detaching from the physical body in pursuit of enlightenment as a precursor to death.[1] An older man would transition from the life of a grandpa to the life of an ascetic, renouncing his home and physical possessions (often including his clothes). He'd wander the woods like a vagabond, beg for alms, and meditate in caves. As with the young boys training for priesthood, yogic wisdom and purification practices were the only thing he had to focus on. Young monks and wandering ascetics had abundant time to memorize, dissect, and embody yogic philosophy. *It was their only job!* They passed down this knowledge orally for centuries. Then they moved to writing it on palm leaves, which weren't exactly created to last for all of eternity, nor were they accessible to the illiterate masses.

This opens up a big question: What guidelines exist for the rest of us in living our yoga? What if you aren't a priest boy or an elderly monk? The answer lies inside a book called the *Yoga Sutras*.

WHAT ARE THE *YOGA SUTRAS* AND WHY SHOULD YOU CARE?

Think of this ancient text, the *Yoga Sutras*, as 196 "yoga tweets": bite-size nuggets of yogic wisdom, pulled from many traditions, millennia old and distilled to their essence.[2] You may have heard of revered Indian sage Patanjali, the consolidator of this body of work. Patanjali did not invent the concepts in the *Yoga Sutras*, but sometime in the misty second century BCE, he brilliantly curated the far-ranging yogic wisdom of the time into an actionable how-to manual. The fact that Patanjali wrote in aphorisms—short sound bites designed for easy memorization—means each *sutra* is highly open to interpretation. This has led us to some interesting places over the centuries.

For example, much attention in the West has been placed on book 2 of the *Yoga Sutras*, in which Patanjali outlines eight practices and ethical principles to lead monks and devotees to the previously mentioned state of enlightenment (*samadhi*). Dozens of modern yoga books can walk you through the details of Patanjali's "eight limbs," decoding these ethical tenets and mapping them to a modern, busy life. If you want to elevate your spiritual life beyond the confines of the material world, this might work for you. However, when I was in my rock-bottom year of personal overwhelm, I did NOT find Patanjali's famed eight-step framework particularly helpful.

In the midst of personal and professional chaos, I didn't need enlightenment—I needed a life raft. In those dark months, my goal was to survive until bedtime each day. Achieving nirvana was the furthest thing from my mind. As I fought with the insurance company for complex medications for my father while sprinting across the room to keep my baby from cliff-diving off the couch, I started wondering, Could yogic philosophy help me? In the midst of craziness and despair? I wasn't a recluse, practicing for hours a day, and I couldn't cloister myself in an ashram. Probably like you, I was a beautiful hot mess of a person with real-world commitments, the occasional crisis, kids, a dog, a job, and clutter in my kitchen and garage. Was anything in the *Yoga Sutras* practical, easy, and doable for me (and YOU)?

ENTER THE SHORTCUT SECRET SUTRA

Turns out, clever Patanjali sneaked in one gem of a sutra for those of us who are not in an ashram or a cave. The majority of us live in a world where our chief need isn't to prepare for the next life but to navigate the complex challenges of this one—with compassionate action. For those of us who need to *act* in the world (rather than *transcend* the world), there is a nugget of yogic wisdom—a *perfect sutra*. It's just overlooked by hard-core yoga enlightenment seekers. To expand yoga's healing brilliance into your day-to-day life beyond the poses, look at the first line of the second book of the *Yoga Sutras*:

> *Tapaḥ svadhyay-esvarapraṇidhanani kriya-yogaḥ*[3]
> Translation: "Yoga in action is self-awareness, transformation, and surrender."

Let's break this aphorism apart word-by-word to discover its magic. Let's start with the final words: *kriya-yogah*. This means "yoga in action."[4] The yoga Patanjali is describing here is practical: a tool you can use, moment to moment, as you face challenges throughout your day. Amid the screams of your toddler while you're stuck in your older child's never-ending school pickup line—*this* is when you practice yoga—in an actual moment that's challenging. This *kriya-yogah*—yoga in action—informs how you move through life, beyond the confines of a sticky mat.

The prior words in this sutra provide a formula for acting in the world with grace and compassion. Yoga in action isn't yoga to transcend life, but yoga to triage the immediate problem in front of you. The best news? It can be applied to everything: your job, your marriage, and the irrational anger you feel when your mother-in-law loads the dishwasher the wrong way.

> **Kriya-yogah:** Yoga in action. Yoga that helps you mentally tackle the hurdles of your day. Not physical yoga on a sticky mat. Yoga that helps you solve the real-world problem in front of you.

Now we know what we're aiming at: an embodied, grounded, moment-to-moment practice of yoga beyond the confines of a mat. The kind that gifts you with an elevated awareness, an inner sense of calm, and an intuitive clarity about how to best forge a path ahead. So what's the formula? That's where the other three words of the sutra come in. Patanjali gives us three principles—three tools—three practices for achieving yoga in action in the remaining three words of the secret sutra:

1. *Svadhyaya***:** Nourishing self-awareness. You must be willing to observe yourself and how you take action. This word is often translated as "self-study." If you don't take care of yourself, you'll be continually depleted and incapable of showing up as your best self. Self-awareness leads to self-care. If you aren't aware of how you feel or what you need, you'll never be happy.

2. *Tapas***:** Transformation. You must be willing to change. *Tapas* is difficult to translate into English. Think of it as persistence, determination, or the heat of your burning desire to evolve. I interpret *tapas* as your choice to transform your habitual tendencies, usually by cultivating the opposite of what you'd normally do. This isn't easy. *Tapas* means choosing to be flexible when you'd rather stay rigid. Or the inverse: creating a boundary when it's more comfortable not to. *Tapas* is your willingness to act in new and different ways, even if it scares you. Yoga in action takes effort and courage. If you're

unhappy with a certain result or outcome, *tapas* says it's YOU who needs to change—your behavior, mindset, or approach. *Tapas* forces you to question how you operate, to experiment with new behaviors, and to strive intentionally to transform your ingrained default patterns.

3. ***Ishvara pranidhana*:** Let it go, surrender. This term is often traditionally translated as "surrender to God." I interpret it as "relinquishing control of the uncontrollable"—of all the people and circumstances that you can't control anyway. This isn't easy, but if you can do it, you get back *so* much energy. The end result of trying to control people and circumstances outside your control is suffering. Let it go. Yoga in action means spending your energy wisely.

These three principles within the secret sutra are a recipe for serenity: a CliffsNotes version of Patanjali's entire yoga philosophy. Hold an awareness of your ingrained patterns, figure out how to nourish yourself, and take transformative action to evolve, all while letting go of control over the outcome, trusting that everything is working out in your best interest. These three skills serve as a cheat sheet for the overwhelmed, for those of us struggling in the real world, trying to find calm and ease in our days. I believe with all my heart that these three principles are learnable. Cultivating the skills of yoga in action is practical and in your best interest. Use them to solve whatever real problem you're facing in your modern life, right now!

FROM STRESSED TO SERENE WITH
THE THREE SKILLS OF YOGA

Overwhelm, burnout, clingy family, crazy colleagues, the computer's hard drive crashing—I've yet to find anything the skills of yoga in action can't solve. I've coached more than a thousand students, each with dozens of challenges, to uplift their lives and find calm, even joy. How? By putting these three skills of yoga in action to work in their lives. Let's dissect them one by one so you can do this too.

Skill 1: Nourish Self-Awareness (*Svadhyaya*)

Instead of "self-study," some translators have defined *svadhyaya* as "one's own reading."[5] Interesting. How well would you say you're able to read yourself? Your habitual reactions, your patterns, your default preferences, your biases? Are you aware that on days in which you conduct four conference calls in a row, you usually end up depleted and fighting with your spouse after work? Are you aware that you tend to obsess over money, just like your mother? Or that conversations about politics can be especially stressful for you? Beyond your mind and emotions, are you aware of your own body? For example, are you aware that when your boundaries are crossed, your throat constricts? Or that anxiety creeps in when you skip a meal or defer lunch to 2:00 p.m.? If so, what do you do with that information? Do you leverage it to set yourself up for success? For example, by pre-ordering lunch the night before? Or do you shove away this awareness and rush about your life in the same well-worn patterns?

Without self-awareness, you have no idea why you're so irritable, angry, happy, or depressed. You're unable to take care of yourself or meet your own needs. This sets you up for failure in every other area of your life. Think about it: If you're taking action from a place of ignorance and depletion, why would you expect *anything* to go well? Without self-awareness, I personally am an impatient workaholic with no time to spare for my family, my interests, or fun. Practicing self-awareness grants me a glimpse at my unconscious, internal operating system and gives me an opportunity to change the script.

The problem? Most of us are experts at *avoiding* introspective work.

We'd rather do just about anything other than witness our default programs. It can be uncomfortable, even frightening, to slow down and
dig into the deeper truth of what's *really* going on inside ourselves. In
our fast-paced modern world, time spent in self-reflection is at best seen
as navel-gazing (productivity being, of course, the highest good). At
worst, it's seen as self-absorption. Instead of investigating our feelings,
most of us choose to numb ourselves with a distraction: we open our
work email, scan the news, or zone out, doom-scrolling on our phones.

Over the last twenty years, the benefits of being self-aware have
become better known in the spirituality and wellness sector, and
they now are well documented by medical science.[6] But what is the
point of self-awareness if you don't *act* on it to change your life for
the better? If my goal is to live and embody *svadhyaya*, I've found
self-awareness has no value unless I then choose to *honor* my feelings
and desires and use them to *practice* self-care.

> *Svadhyaya:* Awareness that leads you to look within, and
> discover the best way to nourish yourself in the present
> moment.

Think of it this way: You're a unique soul. You've been divinely
placed in our world at this moment. You're here to share your gifts
and experience joy. But the beautiful essence that is uniquely YOU
cannot send out its radiance if you're stressed, overwhelmed, resentful, and depleted. Nourishing self-awareness (*svadhyaya*) asks you
to pause your inner monologue of stress, overwhelm, resentment,
and self-doubt (remember that default programming from chapter 1?) and ask the deeper questions: *How do I feel? What do I really
need? How can I fill up my own cup? How can I nourish myself in this
moment? Where can I find joy?*

Practicing self-awareness means getting to the root cause of your complaints and exposing your innermost desires. Once you break through the mind's surface chatter to uncover what you really need, you're able to take care of yourself. One baby step at a time, you move closer to what fills you up.

For example, you might think what's bothering you is your overly demanding boss (and everything that's wrong with *her*). But if you dig a layer deeper, you discover that you actually have a desire for more autonomy and creativity in your role. It's not about your boss. In yoga, it's always about YOU! So instead of staying stuck by complaining about your boss, you take a deep breath to call in self-awareness and discover that your frustration stems from a desire for more independence and inventiveness. You're now empowered with awareness—so act on it. Perhaps you ask for a transfer to a more creative team. Or you start writing poetry at night as a creative outlet beyond work. There are limitless possibilities for nourishment and joy when you develop the habit of looking within—and then honor the desires you find.

For the record, this is not selfish. In learning how to unearth your true desires and nurture yourself, you show up as a better partner, lover, boss, sibling, parent, colleague, and friend. Do not rob the world or your loved ones of the authentic, fulfilled you! Learn how to take care of yourself so you can show up replenished and radiant, with the gift of your highest self.

Consider an example. You may notice you're angry (self-awareness), and as you slow down and breathe, you feel your stomach cramping. You're actually hungry. You have an unshakable desire for food. Stop what you're doing and nourish yourself by making a snack (self-care). Or perhaps your partner's telling you that he never wants to spend another holiday with your family. You're outraged, but instead of fighting back, you take a beat. You look inside (self-awareness) and realize that what you're really feeling is a deep sadness that your two families can't get along. Instead of engaging in battle with your partner over vacation plans, you could express this sentiment of sadness with tender vulnerability. Or you could excuse yourself from the conversation to make some hot tea, take a bath, go for a walk—anything that nourishes you. In these ways, you honor and process your emotions (self-care).

Without self-awareness, you have zero ability to take care of yourself. By avoiding self-awareness (and consequently self-care), you remain depleted and resentful. For me, practicing self-awareness is all about slowing down and getting honest with myself. Ask: *How do I feel? What do I really want? What could I do right NOW that's nourishing?*

You might be thinking, *That's great and all, Brett. But I can't have what I want! And finding something nourishing to do is hard!* Maybe you want a yacht. Or to stop working forever. OK, sure. Maybe you can't have those things. But the beauty of self-awareness is that it asks you to dive deep below your surface-level thoughts. Material things are usually representative of a feeling. A deeper craving you think you'll satisfy when you obtain the object of your desire. If you find yourself really craving something, try to identify the underlying feeling. What does owning a yacht mean to you? What would retiring early give you? When you have that answer, the yacht might still be off the table, but you could probably still meet the need for belonging, success, achievement, adventure, and rest by creatively nurturing yourself in other ways. When you meet that need for yourself, your obvious delight in this feeling can be a radiant gift to those around you.

Experiment! For example, dig deeper into the thought *I never want to work again.* Is that *really* true? With introspection, you may discover that your job is actually fine. The resentment stems from a desire to spend more time outdoors, working in your beloved garden. Can you honor your deepest desire to putter around your yard?

Maybe you could wake up a little earlier each day to dig in the soil. Or negotiate with your boss for flextime, working later some days for a Friday off to gather your rosebuds. Or plan your PTO for planting season so you can get set up for the year ahead. *Svadhyaya*, this first principle of yoga in action, empowers you. It puts you in your rightful place, in the driver's seat of your life. It challenges you to get curious about what lights you up and find creative ways to celebrate and look after yourself. Only then can you embody your unique joy. When you take action from a joy-filled place, the result (and the ride to get wherever you're going) is usually a lot more pleasant.

How Well Do You Know Yourself?

How much time have you spent sleuthing for little ways to nourish yourself? Have you ever itemized the activities that bring you the most joy? How easily can you tell me five things you could do right now that would make you feel like your cup runneth over with happiness? In my Yoga for Self-Mastery course, I work with my students to create a list of one hundred unique self-care activities that nourish them. Start now with twenty.

When were the times that you felt carefree? Childlike? Lit up from within? Were you ice-skating? Doing yoga? Finger painting? Hanging out with your best friend? Use this prompt: _____ *nourishes me to feel safe, happy, and creative.* One student told me that simply holding a hot beverage nourishes her. Another said stroking a pet. It could be walking. Or wearing clothes warm from the dryer. Brainstorm your nourishment list here:

1. _____

2. _____

3. _____

4. _____

5. _____

Life is full of disappointments, frustrations, and sadness. But the beauty of self-awareness is that it beckons you to look within, to examine what makes you feel happy and free. It will take trial and error. It might require some experimenting on your part to figure out what deeply nourishes you. For example, I thought I wanted to join a local hiking group to spend more time in nature. However, on the first hike, the whole group was chatting away the entire time. When I got home, I felt depleted, not filled up. I realized my actual desire was for solitude. A nature walk alone would have been a better choice. Figuring out how to best honor your true feelings takes practice.

At this point, my self-care list includes strolling by the water while listening to eighties music, sampling weird food combinations while my kids are asleep, soaking in a hot bath followed by taking a cold shower, pedaling my bike through the woods, wearing moisturizing hand masks as I read, and singing goofy made-up songs in the car to my toddler. This is yoga in action because these activities are uniquely nourishing for me personally and help my unique joyful essence come forth. These small actions usher me toward my authentic, joy-filled self (*prakriti*)—who I was before my fears, insecurities, and society-taught default thought patterns crept in. Here's how you can do this too.

YOGA HABIT: *Nourish Yourself*

How to do it:

1. **Pause:** In order to practice introspection and identify how you can nourish yourself, you need to *slow down*. Become still. Connect with the star of your life—YOU. I know you're busy. But this is your one and only life. What could be more important?

2. **Breathe Deep:** Take the biggest inhalation you can muster, followed by the longest exhalation. (We'll cover how to do transformative yoga breathing in chapter 4.) This deep breath powers your whole body, not just your intellectual mind. If you listen closely, your body often reveals a quick way to make you happy. You might be craving lemonade. A meal. A shower. Or a five-minute nap.

3. **Ask Yourself:** *How do I feel? What do I want?* What would be nurturing, and achievable, in this moment that matches your need or desire? Get creative.

Pro Tip: You can receive nourishment only in the *present moment*. Ever had a massage but spent your entire time in the face cradle reliving a troubling conversation that happened last night over dinner? It looks like self-care, but it's not nourishing because your mind is somewhere else. Stay present with yourself. Slow down, find little things that bring you joy, and savor them in the NOW.

As you start brainstorming potential self-care activities, you might start thinking: *These are SO achievable! Why don't I prioritize any of these things?* Or the inverse: *What if I don't have time to do anything on my list?* Don't worry. Skill 2 deals with these exact questions directly.

If you're still struggling with the ideas of self-awareness and self-care, the second skill of yoga in action is here to help you.

Skill 2: Choose Transformation (*Tapas*)

Remember your out-of-balance persona (*vrakriti*) from the previous chapter? That Sanskrit word encompasses how you're operating right now: with your family-programmed personality and negative life circumstances adding crusty layers over your true identity. Your goal is to reclaim your joyful, authentic self (*prakriti*). But unfortunately, your unbalanced *vrakriti* wants everything in your life to stay the same. It loves the familiar because the familiar feels safe. This may mean you keep dating the same type of person, or experiencing the same insecurities in a relationship—regardless of who your partner is. Maybe you're always anxious, regardless of what's going on in your life. You might want to change, but you don't know how. Without yogic tools as an antidote, your habitual coping mechanisms will run your life. You won't evolve unless you figure out how to change. Enter *tapas* (not the kind you eat at a Spanish restaurant!).

While *tapas* has a meaning in the actual yoga poses—the physical heat we generate in a deep squat like Chair Pose—its meaning goes far beyond this. *Tapas* is often translated as "internal fire," "discipline," or "motivated, focused energy."[7] Think of it as the heat of your burning desire to evolve. The friction you feel as you take uncomfortable and unfamiliar steps to transform your life for the better.

As Newton's first law of motion tells us, an object in motion stays in motion. The object will keep on its same trajectory unless you add some heat, some energy, to stop it or change its direction. That's how you break old habits that don't serve you and create new ones that do: You add friction and make the effort to do things differently. Even if fear is present. For example: If you're used to always working through lunch, change it up! Get outside for a walk instead. It will take extra motivation and focused effort (*tapas*) to remember to get up from your desk and head outside. But the only way you'll change your workaholic ways is by taking a different action, and even little choices mean more than you think.

Changing things up in the physical world can profoundly change things up in the psychic world too. Making better choices from moment to moment helps you build confidence when bigger moments arise. Changing old habits and choosing to transform (*tapas*) is a muscle. Each time you choose to do something you usually wouldn't or take action in the face of fear, it gets stronger.

Think of *tapas* the same way you'd think of a muscle like your biceps. It won't grow if you don't put it under pressure to strengthen it. It's uncomfortable to lift weights, and it's uncomfortable to go against your current habits. It takes discipline. Luckily, yoga on your mat expands your ability to tolerate discomfort. The physical yoga poses become a place where you practice *tapas* in your body—testing your limits in a pose or getting "comfortable with discomfort" physically so you can then do this mentally. Your personalized yoga, which we'll design in part II, channels this "evolving of self." It encodes new thought patterns into your body and brain to align you with your highest self. This joy-filled version of you is always accessible. It just takes some training to call it forward.

> **Tapas:** Choosing a nonhabitual action in order to fuel your transformation. Changing undesired habits by doing things differently.

Good news: Doing the opposite of your ingrained habits opens up new neural pathways in your brain, helping you shed unhelpful programming. The more you choose transformation, the more flexible and open you become in your mind and soul. Instead of doing things the same way, reinforcing your status quo, you reinvent and rediscover yourself.

This doesn't happen overnight. It's a daily ongoing commitment to yourself. Your out-of-balance persona (*vrakriti*) has likely been in operation for years, making your decisions and obscuring your true self. Yoga is designed to crack open and shatter these artificial outer layers of fear and insecurity covering the real you. Self-awareness (*svadhyaya*) gives you a glimpse of your deepest longings and desires. But it's through the second skill of yoga in action—you choosing transformation (*tapas*)—that you act on these desires by doing things differently.

The easiest way to start doing this is to hold an awareness of your dominant element (head back to page 13 for a refresher on your primary *dosha*!) and cultivate the opposite. Ayurveda has often been called "the science of opposites"[8] because earth (*kapha*) pacifies air (*vata*) and fire (*pitta*)—and vice versa.[9] For an airy *vata*, cultivating the opposite could look like using a journal to plan out the day instead of winging it. For an earthy *kapha*, it might look like going for a walk after dinner instead of immediately sinking into the couch. For a fiery *pitta*, it might look like leaving work right at 5:00 p.m., even though every bone in your body wants to write that one last email. Whatever you'd normally do, try the opposite.

YOGA HABIT: *Choose Transformation*

How to do it:

1. **Repeat This:** "It's safe for me to try something different." Often our unwillingness to do things differently is rooted in fear. Acknowledging the fear, rather than pretending it's

not there, makes this process easier. Take a deep breath and remind yourself it's safe to approach life in a new way.

2. **Catch Detrimental Thoughts:** Many of our thoughts are in a negative and repetitive mind groove. Perhaps you notice you're tired. You decide that it would be nourishing to take a break and go for a short walk. But your dominant fire (*pitta*) element screams the common refrain of: "No, I have too much to do!" In order to choose transformation (*tapas*), mentally *ROAR* back at that detrimental thought, like a fierce mama lion protecting her baby cub. Experiment. Some of my students like to mentally bark at unhelpful thoughts, like a dog alerting its owner of an intruder. Others voice a silent-yet-forceful *NO!* or literally put up a hand signaling "STOP," or even physically shake off the detrimental thought. Use anything that works to catch and silence the unhelpful, reoccurring thoughts that perpetuate habits you know you want to change.

3. **Create an Alter Ego:** Create a persona who embodies the opposite of your dominant element. Then ask what that person would do. And do it. Here's an example: As a fire-dominant person, I'm a workaholic who needs more fun and less structure in my life. To help me think of ways to cultivate the opposite, I invented an alter-ego named Elizabeth (my middle name). She's a grounded, patient stay-at-home mom who has all the time in the world to make smoothies with her toddler (even though it's so messy), read books to her older son (even though it's not bedtime yet), and do Pinterest-level crafts. In moments when I'm overwhelmed and overworked and feel my fire element running rampant, I know I need to do something different. So I pause and ask, *What would Elizabeth do?*

Visualizing her in my mind's eye then opens up the portal to transformation (*tapas*). On a sunny Thursday after school, Elizabeth would probably take her kids on a nature walk. Seeing this, I tear myself away from the computer and choose transformation by going for a walk in the woods with the kids, even though it's so painful for me to put down my keyboard. But lo and behold, once I'm in the woods with my sons, I suddenly find my joy.

When my students start practicing their opposites, it feels terrifying—at first. It feels scary to take a spontaneous day off when you're a workaholic, or leave a huge tip if you're typically frugal. What if there's an emergency? What if you need that money later?

But what's so powerful about choosing transformation (*tapas*) is that over time, it gives you the lived experience you need to debunk the stories you may be telling yourself. It reveals that so many of your fears are unfounded. The email newsletters I was so afraid to send my audience? My fear dissolved when I got clear feedback that people loved receiving them. My fear that people would hate my yoga classes had no basis in reality. You have the right to explore new ways of doing and being—whatever your negative or habitual thoughts say.

Better still, choosing transformation (*tapas*) changes your energy in the moment, often yielding unexpected positive results. After forgoing work and taking a nature walk with my two boys in the above example, I was so mellow, happy, and fulfilled upon returning home that my husband was inspired to keep me in that glowing state. He volunteered to put the kids to bed, opening up extra time I needed for my office work—time I hadn't even been expecting. Once I sat down at my desk, the problem I had been fussing over previously appeared in a totally new way. My perspective had shifted, and so had my problem-solving skills. What might have taken me three hours to solve before the woods walk took only one hour after. Because I committed to balancing my excess fire by cultivating the opposite, I felt happier and more myself, and I achieved more success. The people around me picked up on that radiant energy, so the rest of my evening progressed in a totally different, brighter pattern. What a welcome change!

Pro Tip: Practicing physical yoga on a mat is a wonderful way to practice *tapas* in your body—by testing your limits in a pose or doing a style of yoga you'd rather avoid. If you want to practice yoga in a way that accelerates your personal transformation, the aim is to get comfortable with discomfort. The most potent yoga expands your capacity to tolerate fear and uncertainty, and it's in that space that you create change. Just as Downward Dog might feel uncomfortable at first, so will setting up that dating profile or telling your boss that you're at capacity. In part II we'll craft your physical practice to fuel this evolution. Leverage your time on the mat to draw your most joyful self forward.

Skill 3: Relinquish Control (*Ishvara Pranidhana*)

When I first started filming yoga classes to put on YouTube, I was terrified. Every time I went to upload a new video, I'd cringe. Major internal resistance flooded my body each time I clicked the upload button. But each time I did, I psyched myself up and decided to choose my faith: Faith that I felt compelled to teach for a reason. Faith that the video might help someone. Faith that if I kept going, maybe I could make yoga my full-time career. Even though I felt terrified, I forced myself to trust that some kind of divine plan was in place that would help everything work out in my best interest. Believing this (irrespective of whether it was true) made the *tapas* of YouTube video uploading so much easier. You can use this mindset hack too. It's actually thousands of years old.

Ishvara pranidhana, the last ingredient of the secret sutra, is often translated as "God," "source," or "universal intelligence,"[10] but my favorite is "supreme surrender." Let it go. Regardless of whether you believe in a higher being, this third key skill asks you to relinquish control of your fear and to have faith in a benevolent universe.

> **Ishvara pranidhana:** Channeling the energy you expend attempting to control people or outcomes into the faith that everything will work out. Choosing faith over fear.

The universe is filled with things outside our control. In fact, anything that's not how you choose to breathe is outside your direct control. The more you attempt to control it, the more suffering you'll experience. This is scary to accept. It's understandable that we choose denial instead—and strive to control the uncontrollable.

Millennia ago, yogis realized the pure futility of trying to exert control in a chaotic, uncontrollable world. Instead, yogis chose to divert that controlling energy elsewhere. Where? Toward the only thing they could control: themselves (their diet, their bodies, their breath, and their own actions). When you relinquish attempts to control people and situations you can't control anyway, something interesting happens. You reclaim *so much energy* you can channel into the self-awareness that leads to self-care (*svadhyaya*) and transformation (*tapas*) to uncover your radiance.

Relinquishing control is by far the most challenging of the three skills, because it forces you to confront questions like, Can you ask for what you need without attachment to a particular outcome? Can you express your desires without the undercurrent of control? Can you trust that life will surprise you in a good way?

This surrender (*ishvara pranidhana*) isn't about becoming selfish or passive. Similar to the Serenity Prayer, "God grant me the serenity to accept the things I cannot change, courage to change the things I can, and wisdom to know the difference," it's about using your energy wisely. It doesn't mean you totally give up. It means you put effort toward what you desire and then detach from what comes next. You go after what you want, but don't make your happiness dependent on the end result. Some of the most difficult places to practice this are with your close friends, family, and partner. I tend to think I know best about which nursing specialization my little sister should pursue, the type of job my husband should apply for, and why my mother should downsize to a condo. But in our relationships, control and intimacy are opposites. According to my favorite relationship coach, you can have one or the other but not both.[11] Intimacy is generated from a sense of unconditional acceptance. That's the opposite of control. Sometimes we don't think we're controlling—we're just offering a helpful suggestion! But that's control in disguise. Whenever you have an agenda, there's an undercurrent of control in the interaction, and your loved one can sense it. Have you ever formed a rebuttal in your head instead of truly listening to what someone else is saying? You're not present. You're plotting how to further your own agenda. It's impossible to be truly intimate while also trying to control. And one of the hardest areas to navigate is parenting.

For example, if I demand my four-year-old son clear his place setting and put his plate by the sink, at best he'll feel controlled (but sulkily comply). At worst he'll lash out (and we'll devolve into a power struggle). But if I say, "I'd love this table cleared," and surrender the notion that him obeying me means he's a "good kid" and

I'm a "good mom," the energy of our entire dynamic shifts. In the first example, I'm trying to control him and the outcome and have projected meaning onto the result. In the second, I'm unattached to what his compliance says about our relationship, and I'm just stating a clear desire. I'm choosing faith (*ishvara pranidhana*) in his innate desire to help, rather than my fear that he won't—and what that might mean about him, or me. It's made a big difference.

The more you release control of the uncontrollable, *even if only energetically, in your own mind*, the more people respond to you differently, and the more energy you free up to put toward yourself. The more you make yourself happy, the more you move toward your highest authentic expression (your *prakriti*—the real you!), and the more magnetic you become. You end up getting what you want in unexpected ways.

Patanjali knew the world was a complex, unfair, unpredictable, beautiful, messy place. He included this idea of faith and surrender (*ishvara pranidhana*) in the game plan for yoga in action because he knew believing and trusting in a benevolent universe would serve us *so much more* than complaining and worrying. The hard work of relinquishing control is a heck of a lot easier when you have faith that the universe is working in your best interest. Letting go of control asks you to trust in the benevolence of life, your fellow human beings, and your own secret longings. Yes, do your part, take action. But then release the outcome. Imagine everything is working out in your best interest—and force yourself to find evidence that that's true. Step away when you feel the urge to control.

The best part? Practicing letting it go frees up energy for introspection and self-care, exactly what the yogis mastered millennia ago. It's not selfish to refocus your energy on how to nourish yourself. Show up radiant instead of resentful. It's not "spiritual bypassing" when you put forth effort and passionately work toward what you want but don't make your happiness dependent on the outcome.

In order to show up as your highest and best self—you as a gift to the world—you need to take care of yourself. When you focus on activities that nourish you, you then show up in difficult situations calm, poised, and imbued with grace. In relinquishing control of others and refocusing on your own actions, you become what those around you crave the most: a compassionate listener who is truly present, attentive to them, without a secret agenda. Relinquishing control requires a hefty dose of humility. It forces you to admit you don't know what's best for other people. Does this mean you can never give advice? No! But perhaps you preface it with, "Do you want my advice? Or for me just to listen?" Focus on staying present with an open heart instead of operating from a place where you know best and have an outcome in mind. When you embody this quiet confidence and grace, intimacy flourishes. Your satisfaction with others, and yourself, skyrockets.

YOGA HABIT: *Relinquish Control*

How to do it:

1. **Find Your Faith:** It can be hard to believe that things will work out, especially when your mental chatter is providing ten examples of how they didn't. Our brains tend to skew negative and "awfulize." So it's essential to force yourself to play a mental highlight reel of all the things going *right* (even when you don't feel like it). A student once told me, "No one ever helps me around the house." When she thought that thought, she got resentful. A bad mood took over, fast, like a sudden storm raging in her mind. I asked her to pretend she was in a court of law. "Prove to me, the jury," I said, "that the thought *No one ever helps me around the house* is FALSE." She had to think for a little

bit. Then she said, "Well, my husband did unload the dishwasher last Tuesday." Pondering a bit more, she followed up with "Sometimes my older daughter takes out the trash." When she itemized every remotely helpful thing anyone had ever done around her house, she actually uncovered decent evidence that the thought *No one ever helps me around the house* wasn't really true. Did she still want more help? YES! But after proving to herself that there was documented evidence of things going her way, she was able to approach her family with gratitude, faith, and optimism, instead of a desire to control. When a negative thought pops up that makes you feel awful, ask, *Is that really true?* Then get to work gathering evidence that it's not. With awareness, there may be plenty of evidence of the good in your life. Cultivating faith gives you a foundation of strength from which you feel safe to surrender.

2. **Choose Your Focus Wisely:** What you focus on increases and intensifies. So once you've gathered evidence of the good, direct your focus toward that! Energy flows where your attention goes. If you're focusing on things you can't control, fear, anxiety, and overwhelm will show up pretty quickly. Notice how your body feels after certain thoughts. *How much longer does my father have to live?* is a question I used to focus on constantly. But it was making me sick to think about. I chose to shift my focus: *It's not up to me how much longer he has. All I can do is keep him comfortable and make time every day to spend with him.* This thought made me feel more at ease and confident as I managed his care. It was highly preferable to obsessing over a time line over which I had zero control. If this sounds like brainwashing yourself, well, it is a little bit. But if you continue to focus

on the negative, or things you can't control, the person who suffers is *you*. Yoga is about entering an elevated state of awareness where you have the energetic bandwidth to choose and direct your thoughts, thoughts that serve you! Most of our suffering is self-inflicted by our lazily slipping into negative thoughts. Focus on what's going right.

3. **Repeat This:** "Everything is working out in my best interest." Can you apply this mantra to everything? A traffic jam is an opportunity to sit and get some extra breathwork in. The plane delay means more time to enjoy your book at the airport Starbucks. That business decision you messed up was a great learning opportunity. Even in my father's cancer battle, there was so much working out in our best interests. I had an apartment big enough for him to live with me. He was alive long enough to meet my son. Of course, I could focus on the thought that he didn't get to meet my second child. But when I think that, the person who suffers is *me*. The more you train yourself to wear rose-colored glasses, to trust and receive the good, the more you benefit from feeling safe and interconnected.

Pro Tip: Fear is beneath every desire you have to control. Anytime you feel the impulse to control someone or something, ask yourself, *What am I afraid of?* This fascinating practice helps you uncover your default patterns and mental programs. Once you unearth the root fear beneath your desire to control, you can examine it with neutrality. Often what you're afraid of is totally far-fetched, not plausible, not happening anytime soon, or just not that big a deal. Sometimes your fear is more realistic, in which case it could be helpful to ask, *What's the worst that could happen?* and *How would I cope?* Instead of indulging in worry, use your energy to gain clarity about the situation and think through a worst-case action plan. For me, this often shrinks the fear to a level that feels more manageable.

YOGA HABITS: THE YOGA GLITTER

Patanjali's three principles of yoga in action—nourishing self-awareness (*svadhyaya*), transformation (*tapas*), and surrender (*ishvara pranidhana*)—work together to improve your day-to-day life. Here's a practical example of how these three skills of yoga in action weave themselves together to benefit your life and relationships.

A notorious micromanager, I noticed I had a hard time relinquishing control of the birthday party my husband volunteered to plan for me. Instead of receiving the party as a gift, I started questioning all his choices, from event venue to cake to food.

The Yoga of Awareness empowered me to notice my inner monologue surrounding the party. I'd become controlling and thought I knew best.

- Through self-awareness (*svadhyaya*), I uncovered the fear beneath my need to control: I was worried the party would be terrible if he planned it alone and that I'd be embarrassed in front of my friends.
- Transformation (*tapas*) propelled me to cultivate the opposite: I smiled and genuinely thanked my husband for the gift of this party. I told him, "I trust you completely," even though my inner micromanager was tearing her hair out and hyperventilating. I took a deep breath every time the party came up and practiced...

- *Ishvara pranidhana*, surrender, by choosing my faith that the party would work out exactly as it should over my superficial fear of its not impressing my friends. I relinquished control of the party and of my husband. When I did so, my husband got to execute his vision and feel like my hero. Was the party different from what I would have planned? Yes! But ultimately he gifted me a day that ended up better than anything I could have expected (or planned on my own).

The result? More joy, more intimacy, more peace, more presence, more transformation.

Do you see? In doing the steps above, I moved through my karma. I learned the lesson that it's OK for me to receive instead of achieve. Taking control of the party would have been easy for me. The letting-go part is what I'm here on earth to learn. In practicing yoga in action, I aligned with my authentic, joyful, receptive self (*prakriti*)—the real me! Instead of letting my micromanaging, unbalanced fear-based self (*vrakriti*) run the show, yet again. You can do this too. Put the three habits to work in your own life. Align with your joy-filled authentic self—both on and off the mat. Become aware of how you feel and nourish yourself (*svadhyaya*), move your energy in the direction of where you want to go (*tapas*), and release any expectations about the outcome, trusting that everything will work out as it needs to (*ishvara pranidhana*).

You can practice these skills of yoga in action anytime, anywhere, and apply them to anything. You cultivated the habits of taking a shower and brushing your teeth. In the same way, now you can integrate these Yoga Habits as actionable skills for your day-to-day life. Think of these three principles as yoga glitter—a dusting of wisdom you can sprinkle throughout your whole day, even when there's no mat in sight. In part II I'll share with you even more Yoga Habits that are like subsets, different flavors of these big three, with more ideas of how you can embody them.

Most importantly, start shifting how you view yoga. Instead of practicing yoga to achieve enlightenment, indulge in it as your opportunity to practice these three principles. Think of your yoga mat as a microcosm of your life. Trying a new response is hard, but you can rehearse by trying out a new shape in your body. Standing up for yourself (or staying silent) in a difficult conversation might overwhelm you. But you can practice embodying Warrior 2 on the mat to build up courage and strength. The physical practice of yoga helps you stretch yourself in the world by practicing on a mat first. All of these actions complement each other and create a snowball effect. Getting *on* the mat amplifies your ability to leverage yoga's wisdom *off* the mat.

As you perfect your tool kit of yogic practices, you learn to trust yourself more and more. You feel safer and more interconnected with the world around you. This helps you take even more transformative action (*tapas*) so your zone of "comfort with discomfort" grows and grows. Your highest self ends up driving the direction of your life.

IF YOU REMEMBER ONLY ONE THING

Yoga is not limited to a two-foot-by-six-foot mat. As the *Yoga Sutras* teach us, physical yoga is only a small part of what it means to live a fulfilling life. Assuming you're living in the world (not cloistered in an ashram), the fastest way to evolve your life is through the three skills of yoga in action: (1) becoming aware of how you really feel and finding creative ways to nourish yourself (*svadhyaya*); (2) getting comfortable with discomfort as you experiment with taking transformative action beyond your ingrained tendencies (*tapas*); and (3) surrendering expectations about the outcome and having faith that it will all turn out for the better (*ishvara pranidhana*).

CHAPTER 3

Design Your Yoga Style

Transform Your Life with an Adaptable Yoga Tool Kit

Yoga empowers you to channel your most elegant self and act in the world in new ways. Each of us faces unique challenges based on our Ayurvedic mind-body type. If you have high air and fire, you need more earth. If you have high earth, you need more air and fire. Luckily, everything in yoga—the poses, the styles, the breathwork, the meditations—is a tool to modulate the air, fire, and earth within you. Think of the yogic practices as a supercomputer that empowers you to balance your unique mind-body type. The end goal? You feeling more authentically YOU and amazing. Power yoga in a hot room increases the fire element. Restorative yoga lying down on the floor increases the earth element. But it's not as simple as choosing one yoga style based on your dominant element and sticking with it for life. You need to be able to adapt your practice from moment to moment—because no two days are the same.

Let's get real: It's not as if you come into balance once and then you're perfectly balanced 24/7. You're a human, not a robot. YOU are always changing. Depending on exactly what you eat, your digestion may be fast or slow. Depending on when and where you fall asleep, you may feel alert or exhausted. If you menstruate, you're literally changing each day of your cycle. Same with menopause! Then add in *all* the outside factors: the seasons, the weather, and global, political, and socioeconomic events. Work frustration and family strife.

It's as if every day is an equation: Sleep + Food + Stress + Commitments + Family + Work + Physical Pain + Time + The State of the World = Your Available Energy. My point: Your energy varies each day. Therefore, it's impossible that one yoga class or style can restore you to balance all the time because it will affect you differently each day.

When you show up at a yoga group fitness class, the instructor wants everyone to do *all* the poses, the same way, at the same pace. What happens? Some students thrive while others leave feeling worse. For Michael, rapid breathing exercises may feel empowering and renew focus. For Jenna, who didn't sleep well the night before and struggles with anxiety, this same breathing technique could trigger a migraine.

If you've ever had an undesirable or uncomfortable group yoga experience, I'm here to tell you: NOTHING IS WRONG WITH YOU! Group yoga classes assume that everyone has the same needs, as if we're all C-3POs made of the same parts at the same factory. Many teachers, intentionally or unintentionally, set the goal that *doing* the posture or exercise in "perfect" form is the essence of yoga. But you know by now that this isn't true.

Let's say it again: Yoga isn't something you're supposed to *achieve*. It's a potent tool available to *support* and *nourish* you—to bring you into balance. The best yoga meets you wherever you are, and then coaxes you to your unique state of balance and grace. True yoga takes into account your mind-body type and what's happening in the moment—and moves you toward your most serene self.

This is why you must *personalize* your yoga, deciding for yourself which styles and poses to include in your practice each day. You'll likely need to mix and match yoga styles. That's why the poses, stretches, and breathwork techniques I present in part II come from a variety of traditions. While I advocate for a choose-your-own-adventure style of yoga, I do find that my students have questions about the styles, and I want to honor the intentions of these different lineages. So let's take a quick peek together.

Yoga Styles Demystified

Have you ever looked at a yoga studio class schedule and felt intimidated? Like, what are these "levels" and "styles"? Interestingly enough, the secret reason yoga styles like yin and vinyasa were developed was to interact with your *doshas* in different ways: to either amplify or subdue your air, fire, or earth. I want to unpack how this works so you can see at a high level how the style of yoga you choose to practice affects your dominant element. My goal is to empower you to leverage all yoga styles as you need them. Like a *Project Runway* contestant, you can mix and match, choosing with intention the styles and techniques that pacify your dominant *dosha* and honor the type of day you're living in. Let's demystify today's modern yoga styles and uncover how each affects your dominant element.

Hatha Yoga

The Sanskrit word *hatha* wins the award for most confusing term. It describes *all* breath-based yoga, including heating standing postures (*ha* = sun) and cooling seated postures (*tha* = moon).[1] Hatha yoga (in most parts of the world) is a yoga style in which you move slowly and hold yoga postures for a long time. The stillness and slower pace give this style a balancing effect for all the *doshas*.

Vinyasa Yoga

The word *vinyasa* means "to link breath and movement"—meaning you might move back and forth between two poses, synchronizing the movement to your inhalations and exhalations. In hatha you might hold Warrior 2 Pose statically for five to eight breaths. In vinyasa yoga you'd flow between Warrior 2 Pose and Reverse Warrior. Vinyasa yoga increases air (*vata*) and fire (*pitta*).

Bikram Yoga

To re-create the sense of practicing yoga outdoors in India,[2] Bikram Choudhury decided to heat his studio to 105 degrees Fahrenheit and trademark twenty-six key yoga postures. Fiery *pittas*, like me, are most attracted to this sweaty practice in a sauna, even though it exacerbates our hot energy. Bikram Yoga increases fire (*pitta*).

Ashtanga Yoga

This style became famous for the traditional Sun Salutation (*Surya Namaskar*), which now pervades almost all modern yoga styles.[3] This beloved sequence of postures includes a Downward Dog, a push-up, and a backbend before you come to stand. You perform this sequence again and again, moving on the breath. Fire-dominant people (*pittas*) tend to love Ashtanga's athleticism and progressive nature. But if the goal is balance, it's best suited to people whose dominant *dosha* is air (*vata*) or earth (*kapha*), who need movement and structure.

Yin Yoga

All the prior yoga styles include standing *and* seated poses. Yin yoga is entirely seated. It focuses on the health of your inter-connective tissue, your fascia—the webby stuff inside that surrounds your muscles and bones. This close-to-the-ground practice increases the earth element (*kapha*).

Restorative Yoga

Restorative yoga is a floor-based practice similar to yin, except instead of holding a stretch, you shouldn't be feeling anything—except your body completely relaxing.[4] A sixty-minute restorative class might include only four postures (each held for ten minutes). Much of the time is spent setting yourself up in each floor-based pose with props and cushions so you can surrender. People whose dominant *dosha* is air (*vata*) or fire (*pitta*), who find it challenging to practice surrender and stillness, need restorative yoga most—and are the most resistant to it!

Kundalini Yoga

Kundalini yoga works with the energy body.[5] It's designed to stimulate particular glands, organs, and meridians, like acupuncture in motion. Students perform repetitive movements such as twisting quickly from side to side or doing squats or shoulder shrugs. Kundalini philosophy holds that dormant energy lies coiled at the base of your spine and these movements can channel the energy up toward the brain. It increases the air element (*vata*) since the focus is on *raising* energy.

STYLE IS NOT THE SOLUTION

Most of my students assume, as I once did, that their healing transformation lies in choosing the "right" style of yoga to practice. The problem with this is twofold. First, reading the descriptions above, you've probably noticed you may be attracted to what you don't need. Second, you may get locked into practicing only one style when they *all* have value, depending on how you want to shift your energy on a particular day.

Let's reframe: Each of the major modern yoga styles could be useful to you, depending on the moment. Each works in different ways, minimizing or elevating the level of air, fire, or earth within you. You might be tempted to just pick out a yoga style the same way you'd pick out a dress that fits OK at a department store. But why settle for off the rack when you could have a "haute couture" yoga experience custom-tailored to meet you where you are and unearth your radiance? Yes, it takes some effort to learn how to design yoga couture that's totally unique to you. But the benefit of learning how to mix and match styles is that you'll always know how to balance your unique energy and nourish your unique body, no matter what's going on in your life. If this feels advanced, I promise you it's actually intuitive. The framework I'll teach you in part II makes your decision process easy. You'll create a perfect blend, weaving together each yoga tradition or style in a way that uniquely benefits you. Learning how to create your yoga, your way, is a lifelong skill with exponential benefits.

When I started indulging in this deeply personalized practice, I feared the yoga police would show up at my door. I pictured kundalini gurus storming onto my front lawn like a SWAT team and admonishing me for adding yin poses to the end of my kundalini practice. I thought the vinyasa police might throw rocks at my window for my moving intuitively rather than adhering to perfect Ashtanga alignment.

Is this allowed? I'd wonder nervously late at night, staring at the ceiling. Turning to the history books, I discovered the answer was YES. Learning yoga's core alignment rules has value (and there are hundreds of books about this already). But yoga was always meant to be *personalized* to your mind-body type. There never was a single "right" way to practice. Don't believe me? Let's go on a quick historical tour.

THE HISTORY OF MODERN YOGA

In ancient times (from 5000 BCE to 200 CE),[6] the two groups of people who practiced yoga were young boys training to be monks and elderly ascetic nomads focused on reincarnation.[7] Both sets of yogis had a common aim: to *disconnect* from the physical body in pursuit of enlightenment.[8] For millennia, yogis viewed the body (with all its physical urges) as an obstacle to overcome. Yogis might fast for weeks or meditate on a bed of sharp needles, all in an attempt to transcend the body and achieve a higher level of consciousness.[9] Yoga was not originally about fitness or self-care. When did this all change?

As with so many other aspects of modern life, the change started around the time of the Industrial Revolution (1760–1830 CE).[10] As people's work moved from fields to factories, a new interest in physical exercise emerged.[11] In Europe, formerly niche activities like gymnastics, weight lifting, and stretching became more mainstream.[12] As quality of life improved with indoor plumbing (starting in the 1840s)[13] and electricity (starting in 1882),[14] the average person took more interest in their physical health. Yoga's philosophical and physical beginnings were in northern India,[15] yet the modern yoga poses we practice today are actually Indian yoga postures influenced by the physical fitness renaissance that was sweeping Europe at the turn of the twentieth century.[16]

Check out this photo. Doesn't it look like a group fitness class?

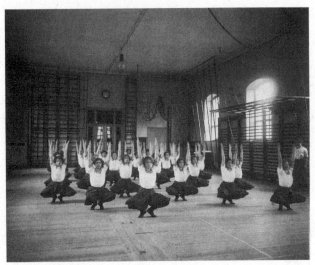

Swedish gymnastics at the Royal Central Gymnastics Institute in Stockholm, c. 1900

Or check out these drawings of American Thomas Dwight performing the exact same postures yoga teacher B. K. S. Iyengar would bring to the West fifty years later.

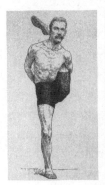
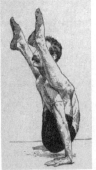
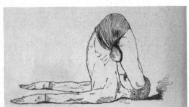

Anatomy of a Contortionist *by Thomas Dwight, 1889*

Or how about this photo from Great Britain in 1931. Doesn't this look like a yoga pose?

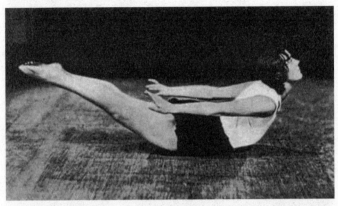

"Seal" posture in the Harmonial Gymnastics of Mollie Bagot Stack, from Building the Body Beautiful, the Bagot Stack Stretch-and-Swing System, *1931. It closely resembles* Salabhasana, *Locust Pose, in modern hatha yoga.*

In the 1930s Adonia Wallace developed an entire exercise method for women centered around stretching and deep breathing.[17]

In the early 1900s, an Indian man saw what was happening in Europe and decided to merge the physicality of European gymnastics with the spirituality of yoga. His name was Tirumalai Krishnamacharya, and he called himself "the father" of modern yoga.[18] Just after the turn of the century, the maharaja of Mysore hired Krishnamacharya to open a yoga center—a prototype for the modern yoga studios we see today.[19] But nobody showed up! In India yoga continued to be seen as something for boys dedicating themselves to spiritual study and for nomads.

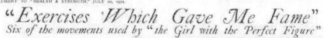

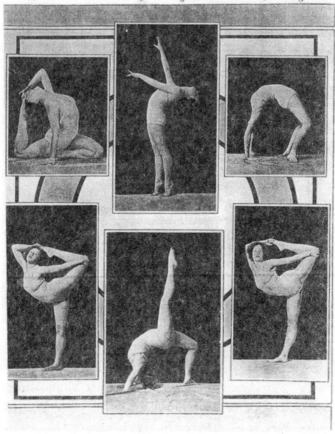

Adonia Wallace, "Best Figure in the British Isles," Health and Strength, *July 1935*

Krishnamacharya had a hard time recruiting students. But he noticed that the types of young Indian pupils he sought enjoyed the Indian martial art *kalaripayattu*[20] and Indian gymnastic wrestling (*mallakhamba*)[21] and were fascinated by calisthenics from Europe. In a radical move, Krishnamacharya decided to blend classical yoga

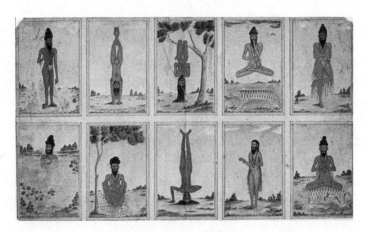

In the Hatha Yoga Pradipika,[22] *written in 1350 CE, there are only thirty to sixty postures, many of which are seated. It wasn't until Krishnamacharya came along with his yoga studio (*akhara*) that yoga became more physical.*

(meditating to achieve enlightenment) with the physical practices of the day. With the maharaja's blessing, he repositioned yoga as a practice for health and overall well-being, ramping up its physical aspects and mixing poses from ancient yogic texts like the *Hatha Yoga Pradipika* with European gymnastics, common Indian wrestling drills (hello, *Chaturanga* push-ups!), Indian martial arts, dance, and contortionism. Lo and behold, young people started flocking to Krishnamacharya's yoga center.[23]

By emphasizing the role yoga can play in the health and longevity of the body, Krishnamacharya evolved yoga from something for a select few (priests and ascetic nomads) to a form of exercise that's beneficial for everyone.[24] The yoga postures we practice today are remnants of his vision and teachings.

At the Mysore palace, Krishnamacharya began teaching different movement patterns and poses to his three star pupils (K. Pattabhi Jois, B. K. S. Iyengar, and T. K. V. Desikachar) based on what he saw each struggled with. Each of these men later brought his own modernized yoga fusion to America. But in Krishnamacharya's style of tutelage, a student learned new poses from their teacher only when they were ready. Jois, Iyengar, and Desikachar's yoga styles, on the other hand, became enmeshed with the American group fitness movement of the 1970s and '80s (hello, Jane Fonda!).[25] Group yoga classes emerged. Yoga brands and franchises proliferated.

In the yoga classes most people experience today, everyone is expected to do the same poses, the same way, at the same time. All the yoga postures are presented to all the students at once, regardless of whether they are ready to learn them or whether the poses are energetically or anatomically advantageous for them. A stark contrast to Krishnamacharya's original classroom in Mysore! Yes, yoga has ancient roots. But it's been in a state of constant metamorphosis for the past 150 years. To me this means you don't have to be rigid in one style. To be true to the ancient understanding of yoga, you must blend the parts that best serve YOU! A baseline knowledge of yoga will give you the right tools for your transformation. But what's essential is to honor your own anatomy and psyche. To discover what works for you as an individual. My goal is to help you turn inward to claim a unique personal practice that serves to balance and transform you. Yoga your way!

If there's one thing you take from this history lesson, let it be this: Yoga is not static. It's been evolving since 5000 BCE.[26] Krishnamacharya transformed the world's perception of what yoga is when he repositioned it as a tool for health and wellness.[27] Each of his students enhanced, evolved, and individualized the practice from there based on his own strengths and interests. The yoga teachers each of *them* trained evolved it further. The idea that we should adhere rigidly to any one style doesn't serve our quest to come into balance.

Are you a history lover? I go deeper into yoga's origins and classic texts in my History of Yoga course at brettlarkin.com/history -of-yoga-course. It features over five hours of lectures with slides and pictures so you can nerd out more.

YOUR YOGA TOOL KIT: YOGA IN YOUR WORLD

Once I took ownership of the styles and poses I chose, even in the scant twenty minutes I had to practice, my whole life changed for the better. Now, instead of contorting myself into someone else's routine, someone else's voice, pace, and poses, I honor how I'm feeling in the moment and adjust my practice to meet and balance my mood. Instead of trying to think, achieve, and follow along, I apply the three skills of yoga in action—nourishing self-awareness, transformation, and surrender—to balance my dominant element and nourish my energy. What this looks like *changes* from day to day.

Over time, just like Mary Poppins with her magic bag of tricks, I've developed my own yoga tool kit of remedies. No matter what's troubling me or how much time I have available, there is always a yoga technique that I can summon to uplift myself.

Yoga tool kit: Personalized yoga breathwork, poses, sequences, and meditations you can use both on and off the mat, in any amount of time, to shift your energy. Yoga techniques that restore you to balance—fast.

Figuring what's in your yoga tool kit takes some thought—and some trial and error. But this discovery process, which I'll guide you through step-by-step next, will pay off handsomely—and save you so much time later on. Why? Because these poses and ways of moving are:

1. Best suited to taming your dominant element and restoring you to balance and joy.
2. Modular, meaning they are totally adjustable. You can do some, all, or none, on the mat or off, as your needs and time allow. This makes them easy to integrate into your day.

Creating your yoga tool kit makes your practice adaptable to your mood, time, and space. Remember: Adaptability creates consistency, and consistency increases your quality of life. The more consistent you are with a physical yoga practice (even if it's between conference calls), the more you evolve spiritually. And if you learn to sprinkle in that yoga glitter (the habits of self-awareness, transformation, and surrender) off the mat, you'll be better able to adapt your physical practice to nourish you in a given moment. It's a virtuous circle.

There's just one last thing to talk about before we figure out the "soulmate poses" in your yoga tool kit: the practicalities of space.

CREATE YOUR HOME PRACTICE SPACE

Rule number one: Let go of designing "the perfect" yoga room or home practice space. This will only frustrate you, slowing your evolution. Plus, as we've learned, yoga is not a space you go to but a mindset you inhabit. Your life is the real yoga studio. And while it can be nice to have a dedicated space, it's not necessary. In fact, I've had my most enlightening moments in the messiest atmospheres.

Like the time I was in India, in my dirty pajamas, doing an online yoga class. My breakthrough moment happened in my tiny hotel room while I was on my own, with my mat crammed between the bed and the wall—*not* in the ashram (ironically!). Or the time I was staring at a tampon wrapper (not mine) in my then-boyfriend's home. I told myself it was proof he'd cheated on me, and I started the free fall into heartache. Then, like pausing a recording, I stopped the plunge into anguish. Instead, I chose to respond, not just react, to the shock. When I implemented the Yoga of Awareness, my chest virtually exploded—not in grief, but in an expansive compassion, a oneness with the entire universe, in a *bathroom*. That's been one of my biggest heart-opening moments to date, even sixteen years later. Not to mention the surprise—unassisted and unexpected—at-home birth of my (impatient) first son. That might be the messiest, most spiritual experience of my life. Bottom line: My *massive* eureka yogic moments, in which I radically evolved as a person, were *anything* but glossy and glamorous. They did not take place on a yoga retreat or in an Instagrammable atmosphere.

What I'm trying to tell you is that practical is better than perfect. You may have judgments about why your current space is unsatisfactory (too small, too loud, too cold, too dark, too smelly, too narrow, too much carpet, no privacy). Become aware of these criticisms—and then do yoga anyway. Adaptability truly is the key.

PROPS TO SUPPORT YOUR PERSONAL HOME PRACTICE

Yoga props are not just for beginners, and they're not training wheels. Anyone can benefit from them at any time. Owning the right set of props empowers you to further personalize your yoga—to make your practice more comfortable, more delicious, and more nourishing to your unique anatomy and energy. Blocks, straps, and bolsters, when used correctly, can help you go deeper into a pose and/or respect your unique skeletal limitations (and differentiate what's malleable from what's not). In my home I created a yoga basket that I bring with me from room to room so I can roll out my mat and all my props *anywhere* it's quiet. (Bonus if I can find a patch of sun.) Here's the gear I recommend to get your home practice started:

Yoga Mat: Think of your yoga mat as your rubberized safe haven. It's where you tune out everything you've been doing in the outer world. On your mat you reverse the flow of your attention *inward* and figure out how to nourish yourself (*svadhyaya*). You know how you can hear ice cream truck music and crave a cone? Your yoga mat can work the same way. These days, when my feet step onto my yoga mat, my mind knows it's time to become introspective: *How do I feel? What do I want? What do I need?* Continually reframing your yoga practice to be about building your safe haven will make you *want* to get onto your yoga mat, even if it's just to sit down and take a "life break" for five minutes.

In terms of brands and materials, it doesn't matter whether it's a twelve-dollar mat from Amazon or a $120 mat from Jade. I've tried them all, and I prefer what's lightest (easiest to roll and carry from room to room) and most practical (grays hide stains really well).

If you don't have a mat or can't bring yours with you when you travel, you can adapt the poses you choose to practice so that the floor works just as well.

Blocks: Do you have a hard time reaching the floor in a Standing Forward Bend? Bring the floor to you with blocks—they're like extensions of your arms. Use blocks in all manner of poses—to support your head, back, hips, and arms. In virtually every case, blocks can relieve pressure on your lower back and enable you to breathe more deeply. Ultimately this means you can truly *relax* into position. It's hard to feel nourished if you don't even feel supported in a pose. I unabashedly use blocks in almost every yoga posture in endless combinations. My favorite is using the blocks in a T shape to support my head anytime I'm in a Seated Forward Bend. Anytime you wish the floor were higher, or your arms were longer, use a block. There are fancy wood and cork ones, but they're heavy. I'm all about portability, so the cheapo foam ones are the blocks for me.

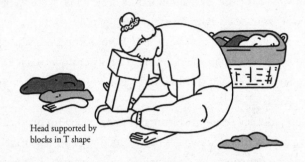

Head supported by
blocks in T shape

Straps: Imagine the teacher wants you to hinge at the hips and touch your toes, but there's just one problem: you can't reach your outstretched foot. Grab a strap, and, as if it were a magic arm extender, you can hold your outstretched foot without having to hunch. Behold your nice tall spine in the mirror! If you're tempted to hunch over and *reeeeaaach*, use a strap instead.

Note: Dog leashes, scarves, belts, and rolled-up towels work just as well as fancy yoga straps.

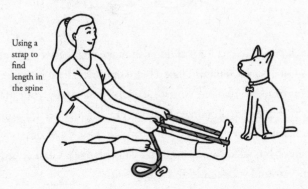

Using a
strap to
find
length in
the spine

Bolsters: Imagine you're trying to relax in a Seated Forward Bend, but your chest can't rest on your thighs. Your spine just doesn't bend forward that far. Solution? Slide a bolster under your chest or belly and ta-da! Now you're supported by a big, delightful yoga pillow. Your lower back widens, you can breathe deeper, and tension vanishes from your shoulders or neck. Plus, there's a built-in pillow for your head. Anytime you see a gap, an empty space in a seated yoga pose, stick a bolster there. If your knees are way off the ground when you sit on the floor, stick a bolster under each knee. If your torso doesn't reach the floor in Pigeon Pose, place your torso on a bolster instead.

Pillows, outdoor patio furniture cushions, rolled-up blankets, and sleeping bags work just as well as professional yoga bolsters. Again, it's essential you feel supported, especially in poses where you're seated on the ground.

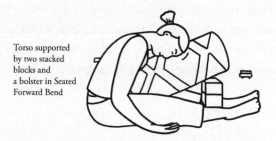

Torso supported by two stacked blocks and a bolster in Seated Forward Bend

Blankets: Blankets for padding can make yoga easier on your sensitive joints. Knees tender? Place a blanket under them for more padding anytime you're on all fours. Does the floor under your mat feel hard? Sit on a folded blanket instead. Having a superstressful day? Pull a blanket over your body in *Savasana*. Don't you deserve to be pampered? No need to buy a special yoga blanket. Grab your favorite from around your home and snuggle up.

Eye Pillow: Why not make your yoga practice feel like a spa day? When you use an eye pillow to cover your eyes, it blocks out external light. This act alone is proven to soothe anxiety and deepen your ability to relax.[28] Eliminating external stimuli helps you draw your senses inward, making it easier to practice self-awareness (*svadhy-aya*). Anytime I'm lying on my back on the floor—doesn't matter the pose—I throw my favorite weighted eye cushion over my eyes.

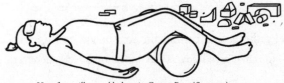

Use of eye pillow and bolster in Corpse Pose (*Savasana*)

Furniture: Instead of thinking of your home as an obstacle to your practice, imagine that every piece of furniture is there to support you. An oversize coffee table is really just a giant yoga block you can rest your hands on as you fold. Placing your hand atop the back of a dining chair is helpful as you try to balance on one leg. It can feel great to rest your elbows on an ottoman while in a Low Lunge or Pyramid Pose. Don't even get me started on walls, which can support your body in almost every pose. My ultimate favorite prop of all: doorways and hallways. Why? Because you have walls all around you to press against, use as leverage in a twist, or lean on for support. Start thinking creatively. Every piece of furniture in your home can be used to enhance your yoga practice.

Gather your props where you plan to practice, or throw them all into a basket, like me. I made sure my yoga basket and my bolster have handles so I can carry them with me from room to room. I also have cheap yoga mats stashed in every room of the house—they're easy to

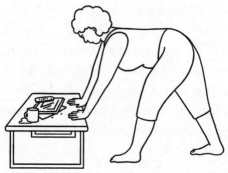

Use of a coffee table to find length in the spine in Pyramid Pose

hide under the bed or behind the sofa or just roll up and lean in a corner—to make sure I have a safe haven on hand whenever I need it.

Want a guided tour of my yoga basket and links with brand recommendations? Watch the full video and download my prop list at brettlarkin.com/practices.

TIPS FOR BRINGING YOGA INTO YOUR HOME

- Keep your mat unrolled as a visual reminder to practice. Place it somewhere you have to step on it (like by your bed or on the way to the bathroom). The more you *see* and *feel* your mat, the more likely you are to get on it.
- Find an online video routine that resonates with you and do it every day until you've mastered it. This repetition helps you learn, if you're a beginner. Good news: I have hundreds of free

videos on YouTube *and* I'm going to help you create your own personalized yoga routine in part II.

- Let your practice be playful and informal. Drop to the floor for five Cat/Cows on your trip from the bedroom to the bathroom. Lie down on your mat for a yoga nap. Dance on your mat while listening to your favorite song. Don't fall into the trap of believing that you should get on your mat only to do a formal class. Spend as much time on your mat as possible, and make it pleasurable.

- Take advantage of the in-between moments. You think you need a studio and ninety minutes, but you really need a floor and ninety seconds. I love squeezing in a yoga pose while the water boils for my tea, while waiting for the bath to fill, and as a transition from work mode to kid mode at the end of the day. Yes, even three minutes of yoga helps your sanity.

Remember, done is better than perfect. You think you need complete silence and special yoga pants, but you really just need the willingness to practice, even if you're in a bathrobe. Kids and doorbells may disturb you. Just keep breathing.

————

Friend, it's time. You know your personality type (your dominant *dosha*). You know yoga's three philosophical principles for taking action in the world. You're familiar with how yoga's main styles affect your energy. Now you know a range of ways to set up your practice space. As we head into part II and start designing your yoga tool kit, it's time to have a DTR (define the relationship) with yourself about yoga. What are you available for? What are you seeking? Let's make this our first practice of *svadhyaya* and get in touch with where you are right now and what you want from your practice.

What's your yoga relationship status?

I'm Attracted to No Movement/I'm in a Relationship with My Couch

You might be thinking, *Brett, thanks for telling me about my dominant* dosha *and these various yoga styles, but I've barely even done yoga. The thought of it is intimidating and there's no way I'm getting on a mat. My embarrassment would be too much.*

Next Steps: Trust that the yoga tool kit I'm offering in part II is unlike anything else you've seen or tried. Don't think of it like a workout or a class. This is all about uncovering the combination of six to eight physical positions that soothe your unique body-mind complex. I'll also offer you more Yoga Habits that have nothing to do with yoga's physicality and are just focused on expanding your awareness.

Remember: In yoga, personalization is what makes the practices transformative for you. You don't need to sweat or do what others would perceive as exercise to do yoga or to reap its benefits.

I'm Attracted to What I Don't Need

You may be thinking, *Brett, thanks for telling me I'm* pitta *and that Bikram is what I want, not what I need, but I actually really like hot yoga so . . . what do I do?* I call this dilemma the "I want to get married, but I'm attracted to bad boys" problem. (It's a problem I used to have, so I really get it!) In life, it's so common that we're instantly attracted to what we don't need. The yoga you're instantly attracted to is usually the opposite of what would suit you best, and it takes time to build the muscle of *tapas* (cultivating the opposite and choosing transformation).

Next Steps: Meet yourself where you are, then transition to what you need. Do whatever helps you get on your mat. Start with the yoga style that you love, but close your practice with one that soothes your dominant *dosha*. Meet yourself where you are, but practice self-awareness (*svadhyaya*) and be mindful that you're not letting the out-of-balance you (your *vrakriti*) run the show. There's no need to force yourself to become different overnight, but you can gently nudge yourself toward what's best for you.

Remember: If your goal is to find balance, unwind destructive habitual programming, and live your dreams, you're going to need to cultivate the opposite (*tapas*) and practice yoga poses and styles you'd rather avoid.

I'm Committed to a Certain Style

You may be thinking, *Brett, I'm taken. Ashtanga and I fell in love years ago, and I refuse to cheat by trying any other style. This is a committed, serious relationship.*

Next Steps: Stick with what you love, but challenge yourself to explore variations and additions that feel nourishing to you. Keep the melody and chorus of your hard-core practice. But just as you might riff on, remix, or cover a classic song, be open to the idea that you could unearth *more* magic by layering in your own personalization elements. If you incorporate personalization tools, the practice you love will become a practice of passion.

Remember: You know yourself better than anyone. With the right tools, adapted to your unique mind-body type, you are your own best teacher.

IF YOU REMEMBER ONLY ONE THING

Yoga is not static or rigid. It's a living, breathing art form, exercise, and philosophy. While yoga is rooted in ancient science, it's been evolving for millennia, and it's *still* evolving—through you and me. The most transformative yoga practice isn't a single style but a set of tools YOU design and adapt to your needs. The breathwork, poses, meditations, and habits you're about to discover will help you overcome real-life challenges, face confrontations with grace, and reveal your most authentic, joyful life. See you in part II.

Part II

Assemble Your Yoga Ritual

Friends, we made it! You've discovered your dominant *dosha*. We've distilled yoga in action into three core concepts: self-awareness (*svadhyaya*), transformative action (*tapas*), and surrender (*ishvara pranidhana*). Your home practice space exists. Now it's time to design the personalized yoga ritual that evolves you toward your most authentic self.

All good yoga classes share common rhythms. If you've been to a yoga class, you're likely familiar with the pattern: your instructor will guide you through a warm-up, then standing poses culminating in a balance or backbend, before you wind down onto the floor. There's a reason for each of these components, and your own personal yoga ritual will share those same five building blocks:

1. SIT: A seated exercise to observe your breath, anchor your energy, and shift your focus from outside to inside (*svadhyaya*).

2. WARM UP: Gentle poses that link breath and movement to lubricate the spine and wake up your body.

3. MOVE: Challenging postures that build strength. These poses flow more intensely and often faster (*tapas*).

4. STRETCH: Seated poses to calm your nervous system and promote introspection.

5. MEDITATE: An opportunity to witness your thoughts without judgment, reprogram unhelpful thought patterns, and channel ingenious solutions to your problems (*ishvara pranidhana*).

Do you see how this framework honors and weaves together the best of each of the major yoga styles we explored? Your WARM UP is rooted in the hatha lineage, your MOVE section leverages the best of vinyasa, and your STRETCH segment draws from both yin and restorative. In the following chapters, I'll walk you through fleshing out each of these five building blocks, step-by-step, to identify specifically what poses and postures best suit your needs. Then, in chapter 9, we'll talk more about bringing it all together. Our ultimate goal: finding the best twenty-minute ritual for you, then learning how to adapt your ritual to the ups and downs of your day—and your life!

Remember, adapting your practice to serve your needs in a given moment is *everything*. This is literally life changing. Without this wisdom, you may be tempted to skip your practice as daily diversions and frustrations pop up. I'll show you how to dissect and abbreviate each section of your sequence to match your mood, energy level, and even time constraints. At the end, you'll have a tried-and-true ritual that can uplift you—no matter how big the distraction, how deep your resistance, or how small the window of time you have to practice.

It's Not Just About the Poses

Let's be real—you won't always make it to your mat. My mission is to help you feel uplifted by your yoga even if you don't have the time or space to practice the physical components. I've included many off-the-mat Yoga Habits that complement the five building blocks of a yoga practice, and I offer additional ways to embody self-awareness (*svadhyaya*), transformative action (*tapas*), and surrender (*ishvara pranidhana*) throughout your day. I'm going to ensure your yoga tool kit is abundantly loaded, no matter the situation. On chaotic days, or anytime you need more calm, you'll have a solution.

Even though I was among the first to run a totally digital yoga business, at heart I'm still a glitter-pen-and-paper girl. I even ship my online yoga teacher training students physical manuals, making sure there are plenty of pages for jotting down their own thoughts and setting their own goals. Why? Because the act of writing triggers action. There is immense power in writing things down. Overwhelming neurological evidence supports that physically writing down your goals actually sparks a change in your brain.[1] With that in mind, I've created this worksheet. Fill it out as we go, and by the end of part II, your potent, personalized twenty-minute life-transforming ritual will be ready.

Uplifted Yoga Personal Practice Worksheet

My Personal Yoga Ritual

Sit (*breath awareness*): _____

Warm Up (*gentle movement*): _____

Move (*heating and strengthening*): _____

Stretch (*winning wind-down*): _____

Meditate (*circle one*):

For Calm   For Clarity   For Compassion

FAVORITE YOGA HABITS

_____

_____

_____

Download the "Practice Builder" Worksheet

Need another worksheet? Want to create extras for different times of the month?

You can download the fill-in-the-blank worksheet anytime at brettlarkin.com/practice-worksheet.

CHAPTER 4

Sit

Notice Your Breath to Change Your Life

"You need to floss more."

My dentist swiveled in her chair, loomed in close to my face, and made a declaration that changed my oral hygiene habits forever: "If you have to choose between flossing and brushing," she deadpanned, "just floss. For your gums, it's actually the most important thing."

Now, you have to understand that, for me, brushing my teeth was sacrosanct. When I worked a corporate job, I'd head to the restroom and whip out my toothbrush at lunch. Yet Dr. Gloria was telling me to bring floss, instead of my toothbrush, to a hypothetical deserted island? I was flabbergasted. And I've flossed every day, ever since.

Why am I telling you about my dental epiphany? Because it's the same for yoga: everyone thinks yoga is about poses and flexibility, but it's actually the breath that matters most.

If you have to choose between poses and breathing, breathe.

In my early twenties, strutting to Bikram hot yoga classes in New York's SoHo, I thought fancy gear and doing the splits were the signs of an advanced yogi. I wanted physical prowess (and to look hot, obviously!). These days, I'm often practicing in my pajamas. From the outside my yoga looks less glamorous, but prioritizing breathing over postures is what activates the deep inner work—the Yoga of Awareness. It's the breath that unveils our resilience, grace, and bird's-eye perspective. I believe that elevated awareness is what we're all really seeking. It's just not Instagrammable.

———

Five thousand years ago, ancient yogis unlocked a powerful secret: To manage stress, we must rise above our thoughts. By elevating your perspective, you can gain distance from your habitual reactions and access peace. If you study yoga's long history, it's blindingly clear that the foundation of yoga was breathing techniques—not physical movement. Even the earliest cave paintings of yogis (such as those in Mohenjo-daro, one of the oldest known cities in the world) depict them sitting in meditation, and scholars are convinced they were practicing breathing. As early as 4000 BCE, what made yoga profound—and sustained this practice-philosophy for millennia—wasn't a headstand or warrior pose. It was mastery of the breath.

As we learned in chapter 3, the physical poses, or *asana*, were added later, expanded upon in texts like the *Hatha Yoga Pradipika* in the fourteenth century, and then popularized in Krishnamacharya's yoga center starting in 1920.[1] The heavy emphasis on poses we see in yoga classes today is a modern phenomenon, stemming from the Western fitness craze that started in the mid-twentieth century. In the 1980s, to take advantage of the group fitness craze, many yoga studios chose to focus primarily on movement—moving through poses for the duration of class. And so the profound power of *pranayama*, yogic breathing, was overlooked, neglected, and even forgotten.[2]

Yoga translates literally to "yoking the mind and body"—the union of breath and poses. This is what brings harmony. But in the West, it often seems that half of yoga has gone missing. It's time to get back to yoga's essence. The good news? We can reclaim yoga's true power together, right now. Let's breathe.

Try It Now: Stop. Take a moment and notice: How are you breathing? Do you feel your breath in your chest, belly, or throat? Is it deep or shallow? Long or short? Moist or dry? Are you breathing through your nose or your mouth? Did your breathing change the second you started paying attention?

Observe for three to five breaths. Simply notice. If you feel pulled toward your phone, or the to-do list in your head, that's normal. If this feels like a mini adult time-out, you're doing it right. If this feels like a minivacation, even better.

Guess what? If you completed that breath observation exercise, you're already a yoga success story. That's right. If you stopped to observe your breath, you did yoga today. And if you choose to notice how you're breathing again later—maybe when you're stopped at a red light, or washing the dishes, or getting ready for bed, or flossing!—in every case, you'll have done yoga again.

Holding an awareness of your breath *is* yoga. Full stop. I don't care if you're rocking a rainbow-shaped backbend or showcasing a five-minute headstand. If you're not holding an awareness of the breath, no matter how fancy the pose, it's not yoga.

Awareness of the breath is your lottery ticket to happiness and freedom. Yoga is the superstar of exercise *because* of this deep body-breath connection. "Sit and breathe" is the first part of your personal ritual framework because:

1. It's the simplest. All it requires is sitting and breathing, something you're doing already (you just add *awareness*).
2. It's the most accessible. Do it from the couch, bed, or car, even for a moment. Then, when the doorbell rings or your cell phone pings, at least you've fit in this most important step.
3. Anyone can do it! If you're alive, you can do this.

Prioritizing how you're breathing, instead of how you're moving, can be a hard pill to swallow. And inevitably, a few pose-competitive students will fight me on this—at first. If that's you, I hear you. It can be challenging to unlearn what you've been taught to focus on. But I invite you to open up to the transformation that comes with trying on a different perspective. Harnessing the power of the breath is paramount, because it fuels your energy.

THE POWER OF BREATH

Are you alive? You can thank your breath for that. Your breath is powering all your major bodily functions, and limiting the breath means quite literally limiting your life. Your most fulfilled moments come from exchanging the most oxygen for carbon dioxide with each respiratory movement.

Just by your bringing attention to your breath, your breathing pattern tends to shift—slowing and deepening. Without your even knowing or practicing a specific technique, and with no additional effort on your part, your heart rate decreases. You may feel more grounded and calmer. Just by *noticing*!

Imagine if all things in life were this easy! What if I thought about my bank account, and then the money in it grew? Or if I let my awareness rest on the piles of laundry in my home, and then it was all magically washed and folded? Or if I envisioned my dream house, and then suddenly I was living in it? Few things happen just by your thinking about them. But this is the mind-bending power of yoga. Simply choosing to *think* about your breath—even without making any conscious effort to change it—ripples positive effects throughout your physiology.

YOGA HABIT: *Breath Awareness*

Anytime you're not feeling how you want to feel, tune out the voices in your head, and observe your breath instead. Ask yourself:

- *Am I breathing fast or slowly?*
- *Is my breath dry or moist?*
- *Do I feel the breath in my belly or my chest?*

Keep coming back to these simple questions. Doing just this, alone, will shift your energetic state. Learn to ask yourself these questions as you pull your awareness down to the breath in your body.

In this frantic world, most of us are masters at suppressing our anxiety, anger, sadness, even our joy. But breath awareness removes the mental trickery we use to deny our feelings. In the stillness of witnessing your inhalations and exhalations, your authentic feelings blossom. Sometimes your feelings may be momentarily unpleasant. You might notice that you feel angry, depleted, or sad. But instead of shoving down these feelings, what if you stayed with them? Observing your breath? Without judgment of your mood or the situation? If you examine each emotion with curiosity and compassion, your breathing provides an opportunity for your feelings to shift and soften. When you acknowledge whatever is true for you in the moment, your perspective naturally starts to shift. You rise above the clouds of your emotions.

Not really a "feelings" person? Try this on for size: Ancient yogis believed that the longer the space between your breaths, the more space you had between your thoughts. The moment between inhalation and exhalation is an opportunity for *pure awareness*. Another benefit of slower breathing with equal inhalations and exhalations is . . . you guessed it: perspective! Increased self-awareness (*svadhyaya*).

Award-winning science journalist James Nestor spent his career studying how people breathe around the world. In his book *Deep*, he wrote about a free-diving competition in Greece:

> After hanging out with [the divers] for months and months, and seeing how they had trained their bodies to hold their breath for five, six, seven, eight minutes at a time, and dive to these incredible depths, I thought if I was going to write about this stuff, I had to experience it myself. The first thing I learned from freedivers is do not pay attention to the watch. Do not pay attention to your depth. Every day your body changes. You stay underwater as long as you feel comfortable. When you want to breathe, you come back up. It is never a competition. The point of freediving is to listen to yourself.[3]

For divers, listening to themselves is quite literally a matter of life and death. And it should be for you too. Reach inward. Observe your breath. Trust your body. This will naturally pull you into the present moment. Only there, in the present, can you cultivate self-awareness (*svadhyaya*).

It stands to reason that when you're stressed and breathing rapidly, you have less awareness, less perspective, less of a chance of channeling peace or happiness. The next time you're seeking an escape route from a stressful situation, or you simply want to exit your own mental madness, shift into being an observer of your breath. Visualize each space between an inhalation and an exhalation, and ask yourself, *How do I feel? What do I need?* The more often you notice your breath, the more your true feelings, followed by your true desires, begin to surface.

EXPERIENCE A FULL, COMPLETE BREATH

Real talk: How often do you find yourself "sucking in"? For many of us, it's almost instinctual when we look in the mirror or pass any store window. That quick glance to check yourself out and *whoosh*—you pull your belly in. If the interconnective tissue in your belly is holding tension due to habitually sucking it in, it prevents you from accessing your full lung capacity. It limits your ability to take a full, complete breath. This, in turn, slows down your digestion and can trigger headaches, pain in the shoulders, neck, and jaw, and even autoimmune diseases. Sucking it in, which many women do unconsciously, could quite literally be suffocating your insides.

The impact of shallow breathing isn't just physical, it's emotional. Taking a short, shallow, belly-sucked-in breath signals stress to your body, mind, and spirit. You're invoking the critical voices in your head to stomp on your spirit. Shallow inhalations high into your chest, with your navel sucked in, affirm tension and anxiety. In contrast, each time you take a full, complete breath—one where your belly puffs out on the inhalation and draws back on the exhalation—you affirm ease, safety, and balance to your nervous system.

This is easier said than done. In order to achieve a full, complete breath, you have to breathe in a way that's anatomically efficient. Just as most of us don't stand in the most efficient manner (hello, smartphone slump), after years of breathing without intention, you may have formed some bad breathing habits. Controlling your breath is how you control your life, so let's take charge together and practice accessing that full, complete breath.

Try a Full, Complete Breath

1. Place one hand on your navel. If you're comfortable doing so, place your other hand on your chest.
2. Take a slow, deep, curious breath in. As you do, imagine filling your belly with air first, and then filling your chest. Ideally, you'll feel the hand on your navel lift (if you're lying down) or puff forward (if you're sitting) *before* you feel the hand on your chest move.
3. As you exhale, think of pushing air out from your belly by pulling your navel in. Draw your belly button back toward your spine, expelling all the breath you can. Engage your core, as if you're doing a crunch. Bring the sides of your waist in as you get all the air out.

This is the anatomically correct way you were born to breathe (before society and trauma retrained you into stress patterns). This full, complete breath is your birthright. If you're not used to breathing like this, it may feel (very) weird and challenging at first. Don't get discouraged: All of those *Whaaaaat?!* feelings are completely normal. We'll do more troubleshooting in a moment. You breathed with this optimal alignment as a wee child, and this skill is available to you now.

MEET YOUR DIAPHRAGM

It's almost funny how so many fitness fanatics are concerned with strengthening their glutes and toning their triceps when the most transformative muscle of all is one you don't need a weight machine to strengthen. Most of your muscles you can see, like your biceps. But your diaphragm is completely invisible when you look in a mirror because it's so deep within you. The diaphragm deepens and lengthens the breath, bringing rich oxygen into the body and clarity to the mind and soul. Your diaphragm muscle is the inscrutable superhero keeping you alive. Let's get to know it a bit better.

Your diaphragm looks and moves like a powerful jellyfish, hiding in the ribs right below the lungs and above the abdomen. It usually just goes with the flow, but—if summoned—wields immense influence. This powerhouse muscle is connected to your ribs, your spine, the muscles in your stomach, and the fascia (interconnective tissue) around your heart and lungs. Expect subtle, body-wide problems if your diaphragm is out of alignment.

Your diaphragm loves unrestricted movement. You know how back in the 1800s, women wore corsets and were constantly fainting? Well, now you know why: their diaphragms were in a literal bind. In an ideal world, as you fully breathe in, the diaphragm flattens down, gently nudging your abdominal organs forward. As the diaphragm contracts and lowers, your belly subtly puffs out. As you exhale, your abdominal organs travel toward the spine, and the diaphragm bounces back up, snuggling under your rib cage.

The fact that the diaphragm moves *down* on an inhalation often feels counterintuitive to my students. When you inhale, it feels like everything goes UP, right? Au contraire—when you breathe in, the diaphragm travels down. The intercostal muscles between your ribs are contracting and pulling UP, making you feel this "upward"

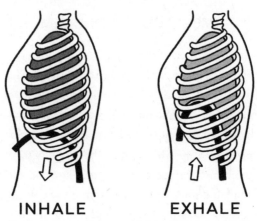

INHALE   EXHALE

The diaphragm moves down on an inhalation and up on an exhalation.

effect. But your diaphragm muscle is contracting DOWN to make room for your lungs to inflate, nudging your belly out of the way.

Why should you care? Because when the diaphragm moves in its full range of motion, you're setting up all your bodily systems for optimal health. When you choose a full, complete breath, you receive the maximum amount of oxygen, getting *the most* out of each precious breath. You're quite literally living life to the fullest.

More than any other muscle, your diaphragm affects the health of your whole body: your emotional state, your digestion, your nervous system—all of it. Anatomy books tend to present the muscles and bones as separate entities, but that's about as accurate as a map showing the world flattened out. In reality, every bone, muscle, cell, and organ exists in a beautiful, messy, unified 3D web of fascia (connective tissue). Just as a tangle in one part of a spider's web subtly distorts all the other threads, a diaphragm stuck in a restrictive breathing pattern can trigger a spectrum of health issues including asthma, shoulder pain, infertility, autoimmune disorders, anxiety, depression, and a slew of other unappealing conditions.[4]

Need more proof? Thank one of the most famous yogis in

history—Siddhartha, the warrior prince who achieved enlightenment through yoga and meditation, transforming into Buddha. Siddhartha was depicted two ways: as Siddhartha, the royal warrior, and post enlightenment with the famous Buddha belly. Buddha's belly is not distended because he's overeating. The puffed belly in ancient art represents someone who is enlightened, a deep meditator who—you guessed it—has mastered the *fullest* possible breath.[5] It's a representation of the power of the diaphragm. The BEST yogis, the Olympic meditators, had rock-star diaphragms, and their ability to move their navel in and out with the breath created a long spine and muscular torso. Of course, there is value in working with muscles in isolation, as you do at the gym. But if you're busy, focus on how you breathe and prioritize your diaphragm. Because of its central location, a healthy diaphragm naturally aids your posture and all other bodily functions.[6] No weight machine or fancy equipment required.

ARE YOU A SHALLOW BREATHER?

If you're struggling to get your belly moving forward as you breathe in, even in a seated position, you may be a shallow breather or chest-only breather. This common condition is called "reciprocal inhibited breathing," and you're not alone. Stress has made most of us shallow, chest-only breathers.[7] If you're a reciprocal inhibited breather, your body and mind are likely not getting all the oxygen they need to truly flourish. It's as if you're underwatering a plant. When the roots of a plant are shallow, it can't fully bloom and grow.

Many of us live our whole lives trapped in a rapid, shallow breathing pattern that—you guessed it—keeps us feeling anxious and inhibits creative problem-solving. A medical study in 2002 proved that shallow breathing is linked to stress and panic attacks.[8] This reciprocal inhibited breathing is also likely a reaction to stressors in the environment. It can happen due to trauma, pollution, or sucking it in to have a flat stomach (please wear Spanx sparingly). It's a vicious circle: Shallow breathing causes stress and stress causes shallow breathing.[9] Over time your body locks in this negative pattern. The connective tissue wrapping your diaphragm and lungs—the fascia—contracts to support short, rapid breaths associated with stress. Taking a full, complete breath may seem physically impossible at first, but it can be achieved with time and practice. Unlike most reciprocal inhibited breathers, you are now aware of it! Which means you're in a position to improve.

If you're a reciprocal inhibited breather with constricted diaphragm fascia, be extra patient. It takes time to retrain your body. Practice the full, complete breathing exercise (page 88) as much as you can: at red lights, in grocery store lines, in boring conference calls, seated, or in bed. All this will help strengthen your diaphragm and loosen restricted fascia. Trust that your body wants to return to homeostasis. It will take time—after all, you may have been breathing this way for decades, and that's a hard pattern to break! But if you keep at it, you will feel the breath shift. Slowly you'll see positive effects blossom in both your physical and your mental health.

THE MAGIC RATIO

For the most profound effect, let's add two more components to your full, complete breaths. First, make sure the full, complete breath is in and out through your nose. Cilia (tiny hairs in your nose—gross, I know) actually filter and warm the air as it enters your lungs. Breathing through the nose is more anatomically efficient than breathing through the mouth.

Second, strive to make your inhalations and exhalations equal in length. Yogis considered the inhalation energizing and the exhalation calming. For optimal nervous system balance, we want an equal dose of each. Enter the magic ratio.

When I was hosting my yoga retreat in Italy, I remember seeing postcards everywhere of da Vinci's *Vitruvian Man*—you know, the sketch of a naked man, arms and legs outstretched, enclosed in a circle. That famous drawing illustrates the golden ratio—a mathematical calculation of proportion that's found in geometry, nature, and the human body itself. The golden ratio optimizes design to be functional and aesthetically pleasing. It's why that simple sketch is *still* so admired. In a similar way, there's a "golden ratio" for breathing.

Here's how it works: You take five and a half breaths per minute (instead of the twelve to twenty you may be unconsciously taking now). These five and a half breaths are made up of inhalations with a duration of five and a half seconds each and exhalations with a duration of five and a half seconds each. Each round of inhalation-exhalation takes eleven seconds. And eleven seconds multiplied by five and a half equals about a minute. Hence the magic ratio breath. The full, complete breath we learned is the anatomically optimal type of breath. The magic ratio is the optimal cadence in which to perform it. This slower breathing pattern signals to your nervous system that you're safe. It shifts your body into a state of calm, gentle alertness. Even if your situation feels anything but safe, the brilliant union of these two ideas soothes your agitated nervous system. This way of breathing is the antidote to your primitive, hair-trigger fight-or-flight response.

So let's try a full, complete breath again, but this time let's do it to the rhythm of the magic ratio.

YOGA HABIT: *Magic Ratio Breath*

Take one full, complete breath at your own pace and settle into the mechanics. Then incorporate an intentional rhythm, slowly. First, on your next inhalation, breathe in for a slow count of three, and then breathe out for a slow count of three. When you can do that successfully, increase it to in for four, out for four. Now try five.

If all of that feels safe, inhale for five, but pause at the top of the breath. Then exhale for five, but pause before you breathe in again. The brief pause is the extra half a second—meaning you're breathing in the magic ratio breath pattern. In the pause you're not breathing at all. This challenges your diaphragm. It's analogous to holding a hand weight motionless in front of you at the gym. Pausing between inhalations and exhalations strengthens your diaphragm.

A quick note: Any one of these counts is a wonderful start. Most of my students need time to work up to the magic ratio. At first you might be able to consistently perform only a three-count inhalation and a three-count exhalation, with no pause at all. That's OK! Keep practicing, and try to breathe like that throughout your day, anytime you remember. Your nervous system is benefiting from *any* attempt to observe or slow your breath. Any effort counts. It all adds up. Practice is better than perfect.

How do you feel after that exercise? Do you prefer to breathe slowly or fast? Or, to put it another way, do you prefer to *live* slowly or fast? Do you want to calmly savor each moment? Or do you want to anxiously huff and puff your way through life?

Legends say cave-dwelling yogis often lived to be 110 years old. Ancient yogis believed that each of us has a set number of breaths in each lifetime. You may have seen images of ancient yogis doing headstands. Believe it or not, this wasn't to show off their physical strength. Yogis loved headstands because being upside down slows down the heart rate. A slower heart rate means you can take fewer breaths per minute. There are yogis today who can extend each inhalation to thirty seconds and each exhalation to thirty seconds. Their diaphragms are crazy strong and their lung capacities superbly high. That's only one breath per minute! This process of taking only the breaths you truly need aims to *literally* extend your life span. Hanging upside down to slow your breath rate and heart rate is great antiwrinkle therapy too.

YOUR BREATH AND EMOTIONS ARE IN A RELATIONSHIP

Ever see those wall-mounted Nest Thermostats that digitally showcase the temperature of a house? (I was totally psyched when I finally could afford one.) With a quick tap you can turn on the heat or AC and program your house to suit your immediate needs. Well, centuries ago, yogis discovered they could control their "body houses" through breathing patterns called pranayama. Depending on the cadence, interval, orifice (nose or mouth), and rhythm with which they chose to breathe, they could control the thermostat to make their bodies more alert or more relaxed.

Full, complete breathing is the essential foundation of your personal breathing practice, but there is so much more to explore. Breathing through your nose or mouth, switching nostrils, emphasizing and elongating your inhalation or exhalation—all these are tools you can use to communicate with your nervous system and change your emotional state.

You already know on an intuitive level that your breath reflects your emotions. When you're freaking out, what does your best friend always say? "Take a deep breath." In the movies, if a character is taking short, shallow breaths, you know they're anxious. They know the villain is lurking around the corner. If someone is sighing, you know they feel tired or sad. Someone flaring their nostrils is angry, ready to lash out. Ever watch your child or significant other fast asleep? Their breath is slow and deep, transporting them to peace. So sweet to see such utter relaxation!

The best part of this breath-emotion connection? It doesn't have to be a vicious circle. You can use your thoughts and emotions to positively alter your breath, and you can use your breath to influence and change your thoughts and emotions. It sounds surreal, but this is scientific reality.

Your emotions and your breath are in a reciprocal relationship, the ultimate power couple. Think of them like Beyoncé and Jay-Z, Michelle and Barack Obama, Meghan and Prince Harry. Your emotions and your breath work together. They mirror each other. That's why pausing to notice your breath clues you in on your emotional state. This is amazing news. Why?

Your breath has the power to influence your emotions. Meaning your breath is like a divine dial—an invisible lever—to access your inner universe. What's astonishing: Your breath can regulate your nervous system. If you breathe with intention, you can control your mood: access calm, ignite your energy, channel your dreams, or brainstorm your goals. All with your breath. Rather than just accepting your current breath pattern and a nervous system that might be agitated, you have the power to *change* the situation. When every cell in your body is flashing "anger," you have the power to flick the switch and choose a breath pattern that de-escalates your system. Conversely, if you're feeling sad and lethargic, you can choose to breathe in a way that invigorates you, boosting your energy and spirit. No matter what you're feeling or needing, you can pull a yogic breathing technique out of your yoga tool kit and change the state of your nervous system. If only these skills were taught in school!

YOGA HABIT: *Sigh It Out*

Most of us have a habitual bracing pattern—an ingrained physical response to stress that is triggered anytime anxiety creeps in. I begin to hold my breath and elevate my shoulders slightly. Other common stress tells include nail biting, lip licking, glute tensing, chin dipping, fidgeting, and grabbing your phone for distraction. I challenge you to identify yours.

Then, the next time you experience your stress tell, administer the antidote. First, inhale fully through the nose (try to puff the belly out, full, complete breath style). Then, for this particular exercise, exhale through the mouth, stretching your jaw wide and softening your neck. Let out a long audible *siiiiiigh*. Make it BIG. Like a cartoon character sighing. Now do this three more times.

Sighing is such a great hack! It slows down your exhalation, and slower exhalations serve to regulate your nervous system. You override however you may be feeling in the moment with a clear directive to your nervous system to relax. Even better, after each sigh out through the mouth, you're set up for a fuller, richer inhalation through the nose.

If someone glances your way or asks, "Why the sigh?" you can just *siiiiiigh* again and smile. Say, "I'm just feeling so happy and relaxed." Even if you aren't—yet. A series of long, slow exhalations through the mouth means you'll feel lighter soon.

UPLEVEL YOUR BREATH

Extending the exhalation and choosing to exhale through the mouth are beautiful ways yogis intentionally use the breath to hack their nervous systems. In changing your breath, you change your physiology and your mindset. This is just the tip of the iceberg. Breath control (pranayama) is the profound yogic science of changing *how you feel* through breathing patterns. There are literally hundreds of delicious pranayama techniques in yoga. On the following pages you'll find six of my personal favorites. I chose these six because together they target a vast array of emotional needs. No matter the crisis, you can empower yourself through one of these techniques. Just as you have a favorite pair of leggings you wear most of the time, you'll discover that one of these breathing exercises soothes your dominant *dosha* most of the time. That's the technique you'll want to circle and place at the top of your personal practice worksheet.

First, experiment! This is a breath buffet. Experience them all. Notice how each breath technique affects your unique energy. If you're uncertain which breath pattern might be best for your personal ritual, the quiz on page 107 can narrow it down.

Before practicing each breathing exercise, check in with your energy to establish a baseline. I call this creating a frame for your experience. Notice how you feel before you start. Call to mind some words that best describe your emotional state. Observe where you feel the most *energy* in your body (buzzing in your brain, humming low in your belly, tingling in your arms or legs). Then perform one of the pranayama techniques for three to five minutes (longer is OK too, if you're feeling it) and challenge yourself to sit for an extra minute or three to bathe in the afterglow. Each time, ask yourself the same questions afterward—*What words would I use to describe my emotional state? Where do I feel the most energy in my body?*—and compare the answers. Do you feel different from before the exercise? Do you notice a shift in your mood or in your body's energy? Do you feel more alert? Grounded? Relaxed?

Need a walk-through? Download video guides and bonus tips for each pranayama technique at brettlarkin.com/practices.

---

1. Taco Breathing or *Sitali/Sitkari*—Calming

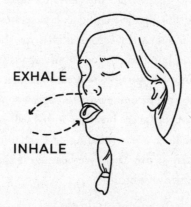

Taco breathing works with an open-mouthed inhalation that is cooling and calming (making it ideal for fiery *pittas*). Use this breath anytime you're overheating, angry, or just in need of some chill. It's also handy when you want to soften your outlook, tap into your feminine energy, or take a break from thinking about your goals and ambitions.

- Curl your tongue into a taco shape so the left and right sides are higher than the middle. Stick your U-shaped tongue out slightly. Inhale through an O-shaped mouth. Let the air feel cold as it rushes over your tongue and teeth. (This type of breath is known as *sitali*.)
- Exhale slowly through your nose. Repeat.

If you are among the many who can't curl the tongue: bring your teeth almost together instead and think of taking a long sip of air in, as if through an imaginary straw. You want to feel cool air over your tongue. (This type of breath is known as *sitkari*.)

2. Darth Vader Breath or *Ujjayi*—Focusing

Ujjayi in Sanskrit means "one who is victorious," and that's how you'll feel after practicing the technique. It generates heat and focus, making it ideal for our earthy *kaphas*. It gifts you the energy of purpose and direction but anchors you in an expansive state of calm. Use this breath anytime you need to hone your focus, stay calm, and solve problems. I often recommend it to yogis who want to work on their magic ratio, because the breath is audible. This gives you clear feedback on how long you're inhaling and exhaling. Occasionally this breathing exercise can cause overheating. If that happens, you can stop and practice taco breath.

- Gently contract the muscles of the throat, as if you wanted to whisper or fog up a mirror.
- Try breathing out of an open mouth as if you were cleaning your glasses, making an audible *hah* sound.
- Practice inhaling the same way, making a *hah* sound. It should sound as if you're breathing like Darth Vader.

- Once you've got the hang of this, close the mouth and continue breathing with this slight constriction of the throat.
- Listen for the oceanic sound (the sound you hear within a seashell) as you continue to breathe with your mouth closed. So still a Darth Vader sound, just way more subtle.
- If you get stuck, try covering your ears to better tune in that inner sound of the breath along your vocal cords.

3. Three-Part Breath or *Krama*—Rejuvenating

Here's a twist on the full, complete breath that helps retrain your diaphragm toward anatomical efficiency. It's nourishing for all three *dosha* types because it's soothing and draws your attention inward. This is a great way to take your diaphragm to the gym if you're a reciprocal inhibited breather.

- Challenge yourself to deeply inhale, pausing three times as you fill up with breath.
  - Inhale into your low belly, expanding it. *Pause.*
  - Inhale into your ribs and back body, filling up laterally. *Pause.*
  - Inhale into your collarbones and chest, taking in as much air as you can. *Pause.*
- Exhale and let all that air go in one long, smooth breath.

In this exercise I like to visualize my torso as a glass, and my inhalation as water. I imagine filling the glass of my torso a third of the way, then another third, and then all the way as I inhale into each area. As I exhale, I imagine all the water draining out as I surrender and relax.

How to counteract reciprocal inhibited breathing: Lie down in bed and place a book or small pillow on your belly. Practice inhaling so the book/pillow moves up in space toward the ceiling each time you breathe in and down toward the bed each time you breathe out. Dividing each inhalation into three equal parts (belly, ribs, then chest) is optional. This exercise is ideal to help you regain a full, complete breath. Placing a book or pillow on your navel and sensing if it physically moves UP helps you strengthen your diaphragm. Continue for three to five minutes or more. Bonus: This is deeply relaxing and can help you fall asleep effortlessly.

4. Alternate-Nostril Breath or *Nadi Shodhana*—Clarifying

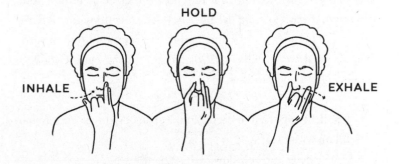

Alternate-nostril breathing is balancing for all three *doshas*. It's designed to harmonize your energy. Inhaling through your right nostril stimulates the left hemisphere of the brain; inhaling through your left nostril stimulates the right. By stimulating both your left and right brains, you achieve a spiritual and physical balance and gain creative insights. This alternating pattern is ideal if you want to elevate your perspective and activate your intuition. This technique coaxes your mind into a focused relaxation during which new insights often bubble to the surface. I first learned this technique while studying in India. My teacher assigned it to me to lessen my relentless fidgeting during the morning meditation (I was struggling to focus). Anytime you feel as if you can't settle down to meditate, mentally floss your brain with this breathing technique for three minutes first. If you have a stuffy nose or don't like touching your face, try armpit breathing (below) instead.

- Tuck the first two fingers of your right hand into your palm, with thumb, ring, and pinky fingers extended.
- Place your thumb just above your right nostril and your pinky and ring finger just above your left nostril.
- Block your left nostril with the pinky and ring finger and inhale through your right nostril.
- Pause, dip your chin, and block both nostrils.
- When you are ready, allow your chin to slightly lift and exhale through the left nostril, blocking the right nostril with your thumb.
- Inhale through the left nostril, hold and block both, and retain the breath. Lift your pelvic floor up and in.
- Exhale through your right nostril.

Once you get the hang of alternate-nostril breathing, add your magic ratio breath—a five-and-a-half-second inhalation and a five-and-a-half-second exhalation, or whatever count feels soothing for you. You never want to feel out of breath. Once you gain confidence, layer in a longer pause at the top of each inhalation and visualize light at the center of your brain. Treasure the total stillness that exists at the top of the inhalation before you exhale and release.

5. Armpit Breath or *Padadhirasana*—Healing

This breath technique balances the nervous system much like alternate-nostril breathing, but it doesn't require touching the face or alternating nostrils. This makes it an ideal alternative for those of us who have a deviated septum, allergies, or just a stuffy nose. Believe it

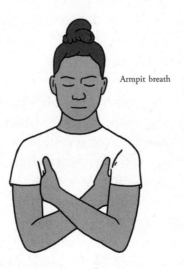

Armpit breath

or not, your armpit has a concentration of nerves that communicate with your nervous system. It's like a magic trick: If you place one hand under your opposite armpit, you change which nostril is dominant. Axillary lymph nodes in your right armpit stimulate the left nostril and vice versa. Keep this in mind the next time you have the flu. If your right nostril is stuffy, practice *padadhirasana* with your left forearm on top of your hand to put extra pressure on your left armpit. To unblock your left nostril, do the reverse.

- Cross your arms over your chest and place your hands under your armpits, thumbs up. (The bottom arm will experience a little more pressure than the top arm, so be aware of this.)
- Close your eyes and take five to ten full, complete breaths, inflating the belly, then the chest. Exhale fully.
- Uncross your arms and then switch which arm is under and which is over, then take five to ten more full, complete breaths for a balancing effect.

6. Breath of Fire or *Kapalbhati*—Energizing

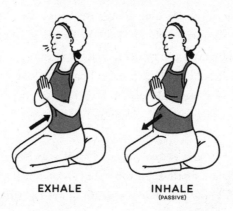

EXHALE   **INHALE**
                    (PASSIVE)

Breath of fire is energizing, heating, and detoxifying. This rapid-breathing technique increases the oxygen in your system, making it especially good for the earthy *kaphas*. Choose this if you want to kick-start your energy without caffeine. Bonus: This breath has the added benefit of simultaneously toning your abs and stimulating your digestion. Avoid doing this exercise while pregnant (see FAQ on page 111).

- Take a full, complete breath—inhaling deeply and exhaling completely—before you begin.
- Now inhale halfway and forcibly exhale through the nose while drawing your navel back to your spine. Continue to focus only on this sharp exhalation (the inhalation is passive). Keep pumping your navel back into your spine to exhale, like a powerful drumbeat. Think *squeeze, release, squeeze, release* as you use the abs and the muscles of the pelvic floor to create a forceful exhalation through the nostrils.

- Continue for one to three minutes. Make sure the exhalation is powered by the navel snapping back toward your spine. Strive to make this an abdominal exercise. Your belly should "dance" as you contract the abs and pull the navel back on each exhalation and release and relax on each inhalation.
- To close, hold the breath in and pause as long as is comfortable after a deep inhalation. Then take several full, complete breaths to recover and recalibrate.

Remember to go at your own pace. Faster is not better! Your body-powered exhalations through the nose can be quick OR slow and steady. You'll know you're doing breath of fire right if your abs are slightly sore afterward. If you haven't been visiting the pranayama air gym regularly, don't overdo this technique. It's better to perform it slowly with proper form, ensuring your exhalation is powered by your navel, than to do the breath only with your nose. Do interval training to work up to performing this breath for three minutes! Pump the belly for one minute, then take a one-minute rest. Work your way up to three minutes on, three minutes off. Make five minutes your long-term goal. Your energy—and mood—will soar!

ASSEMBLE YOUR RITUAL

Grab your worksheet because it's time to fill in the first section: "SIT (*breath awareness*)." This is the most important section because it may be all you do some days! Really! If you're short on time, skip the postures and just make time to breathe.

Select one of the breathing exercises from above to open your personal yoga ritual (and yes, you can always just start with a full, complete breath). Still not sure which to choose? Try this quiz.

Quiz: Sit—How Do You Tend to Breathe?

1. What was your dominant *dosha* from chapter 1?
   a. *Vata* (air)—I love to get creative!
   b. *Pitta* (fire)—I tend to have laser-sharp focus.
   c. *Kapha* (earth)—I often struggle to motivate myself and wish I had more energy.
2. What time of day are you generally planning to practice?
   a. Noon—I want a midday break.
   b. Morning—I want to start my day off right.
   c. Night—I'm too busy during the day, so before bed is best.
3. Do you tend to have a stuffy nose?
   a. Always!
   b. No, I don't tend to be stuffy unless I'm sick.
   c. Sometimes. My sinuses are tricky.
4. Without overthinking it, how would you define your day-to-day breathing pattern?
   a. Short, quicker breaths, because I'm excited or rushing.
   b. I mostly inhale and exhale through my nose when I'm focused (or annoyed!).
   c. I tend to take relaxed belly breaths. Rapid breathing is not my style.
5. How would you most like to shift your energy?
   a. I want to stop feeling anxious. I want to feel more calm and grounded.
   b. I want a higher perspective, no more sweating the small stuff.
   c. I want to stop procrastinating and feel naturally motivated and happy.

Quiz Results

If you got many a's, you tend to breathe in your upper ribs and chest and may be a reciprocal inhibited breather. For you, slowing and deepening your breath is key. Work with three-part breath (*krama*), full, complete breath, or armpit breath (*padadhirasana*) to soothe your mind and help your diaphragm regain its full range of motion.

If you got many b's, instead of using the full range of your diaphragm to get the most anatomically efficient breath, you're trapped in a medium range of motion. This results in a faster breath rate, with the breath trapped in the midlungs instead of getting pulled all the way down into the lower lungs. This faster breath rate can cause overheating, irritation, and impatience. To cultivate the opposite, practice cooling taco breaths (*sitali/sitkari*) and alternate-nostril breathing (*nadi shodhana*) to bring in fresh perspectives. Work with three-part breaths (*krama*) in bed at night to help train your diaphragm to contract in its full range of motion.

If you got many c's, your tendency is to breathe more slowly. This is good, but in excess it can lead to lethargy. To invite in more energy, try breath of fire (*kapalbhati*), Darth Vader breaths (*ujjayi*), or alternate-nostril breathing (*nadi shodhana*).

All of these breathwork techniques serve to strengthen your diaphragm, influence your nervous system, and create space for your true feelings to emerge. More often than not, they'll pave the way to a new perspective. One is not inherently better than another, so choose the technique that best suits *you* for your personal ritual. In the case of a close call or tie, try both for one week and observe how you feel before and after each of your winning techniques. Which shifts your energy in a way that feels nourishing? Remember, your personal ritual framework is designed to *adapt*. Consistency is important, but life throws us curveballs. You can always switch your opening breathing technique based on what best fits you today. Just as you might swap your work-from-home sweats for a suit on the day you're presenting to a boardroom of executives, you might switch your breathing technique depending on the time of day and how you want to shift your energy.

FAQ

How long do I have to do a breathing technique for it to affect my nervous system?

Every moment counts. Remember: Just observing your breath, without even doing any of the techniques presented here, already benefits your nervous system. But for a more profound energetic effect, strive to practice pranayama for three to eleven minutes as part of your ritual, with eleven minutes being a triple gold star. Anywhere in between is also great.

Does it matter what time of day I do these techniques? I've heard I shouldn't do breath of fire at night.

Coax yourself into a full, complete breath all the time, anytime. However, the six specific pranayama techniques above are designed to affect your energy—and they work. Since breath of fire (*kapalbhati*) increases fire (*pitta*) and energizes you, it may not be the one to help you fall asleep. Three-part breath (*krama*) might be a better choice before bed.

What if I get dizzy or light-headed as I practice breathing?

Don't panic. It's totally normal to feel spacey when first embarking on your pranayama journey. You're likely taking in far more oxygen than you're used to, especially as you start practicing full, complete breaths. Whenever you get light-headed, take a break. Lie down on the floor with your calves on a chair or with your legs up on the wall, elevating your feet above your head. Explore a more grounding breathing technique like armpit breathing (*padadhirasana*) instead.

I find myself starting to yawn whenever I practice pranayama and deepen my breath. What's the deal?

Physiologically, a yawn is like a slow, juicy extra inhalation and exhalation through the mouth, initiated by your body. Lengthening your breath activates your parasympathetic nervous system, aka your "rest and digest" mode, resulting in you feeling calmer. So if you find yourself yawning as you practice pranayama—hooray! You and your body are in sync and starting to relax.

Does it matter whether I breathe sitting or lying down?

You can perform breathwork in either position. Seated is preferable for any technique for which you're using your hands (like alternate-nostril breathing). But if you're super tired, you can do mental alternate-nostril breathing (*nadi shodhana*) lying down: Visualize light going in one nostril and out the other.

Anytime you're seated, make sure your spine is long and that your low back isn't rounding. Ensure your hips are higher than your knees (this helps avoid pins and needles in your legs and feet). I like to sit on the edge of a cushion or pillow, elevating my hips. You could alternatively sit with your back against a wall for support. This gets you used to sitting with an elongated spine. Breath of fire (*kapalbhati*) and Darth Vader breath (*ujjayi*) tend to work best seated.

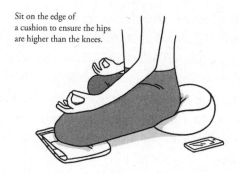

Sit on the edge of
a cushion to ensure the hips
are higher than the knees.

Is it true what I've heard, that breathwork can trigger trauma that's stored in my body? I'm a little freaked out.

If you're healing from trauma, focus on cooling breaths like taco breathing (*sitali/sitkari*) or a three-count full, complete breath instead. Avoid Darth Vader breath (*ujjayi*), and breath of fire (*kapalbhati*). These breaths create energy and heat and can be triggering. Remember, you're in charge. You can always pause any breathing technique, check in with yourself, and stop if needed. There are wonderful trauma-informed breathwork practitioners out there if you crave extra support.

I've heard I shouldn't do breath of fire on my period or if I'm pregnant. Is that true?

Breath of fire (*kapalbhati*) creates heat and lifts energy upward, which is a good thing. But on your period, the natural intelligence of your body is moving energy downward to shed the uterine lining. Breath of fire moves energy UP your body, the opposite of what your body is trying to achieve when you're on your cycle. Yogic wisdom suggests avoiding breath of fire on the heaviest days of your period for this reason. That said, the advice to avoid breath of fire while menstruating is only an energetic recommendation, not a physical one.

Pregnant women tend to run hot, making the cooling taco breath (*sitali/sitkari*) a better fit than breath of fire. After the first trimester, it's wise to avoid intense abdominal workouts that could increase diastasis (which happens when the rectus abdominis—your six-pack ab muscles—separate during pregnancy from being stretched). Since breath of fire powerfully engages the abdominal muscles, it's best to hold off. After you've given birth, return to breath of fire as a highly effective core strengthener—but please get clearance from your doctor first.

What if my nose is stuffy or I have allergies or a deviated septum?

I feel you! I too have a deviated septum. It's very common. Armpit breathing (*padadhirasana*) is a great option. You can also always visualize doing alternate-nostril breathing (*nadi shodhana*) too—it works! Here's exactly what I do when it's time to breathe and my nose is stuffy:

1. Place a box of tissues near your mat.
2. Do breath of fire first to clear out the mucus (this is very effective—watch out!).
3. Do alternate-nostril breathing *after* you've done breath of fire.

Personally, I usually wake up stuffy, and my sinuses tend to clear throughout the day. So I skip alternate-nostril breathing in the a.m. (I do taco breathing instead). I perform alternate-nostril breathing only if I happen to be practicing at lunch, in the late afternoon, or before bed. Are you starting to see how everything is adaptable? With just a little bit of awareness, you can orchestrate the ideal practice for you at any given moment.

You're on your way—breath is the foundation of your opening ritual. Breathing is the most adaptable tool in your kit, since you can do it anywhere. I've been known to pop into a public restroom and do taco breathing. My friend Kate does mental alternate-nostril breathing in her car at stoplights. Speaking of...

YOGA HABIT: *Park and Breathe*

Want to know my favorite place to slip in my daily breathing practice? The car! When I pull into my garage, I close my eyes and take a moment to indulge in some full, complete breaths. I choose to indulge in this magic limbo, a time when I'm between worlds. I know that once I go into the house, I'll inevitably have to do something, so I prioritize my mental health and snag some solitude first.

Taking these in-between moments, the transitions in your day, is an easy way to gift yourself time for a pranayama practice—and begin reaping the profound rewards. Rather than reaching for your phone, reach for your yoga tool kit. Place a hand on your navel and do a few full, complete breaths or a technique of your choice. Practice it while you're on the bus, train, or subway. Or while you're in line at the doctor's or dentist's. Or while you're waiting for the water to boil, the dryer cycle to stop, the on-hold phone Muzak to end. You'll find dozens of opportunities.

IF YOU DO ONLY ONE THING

Observe your breath throughout your day-to-day life. On the phone, at your desk, cooking a meal—pause and notice. Close your eyes and invite in a full, complete breath, even if it's just for a few seconds. Even if you think you're doing it wrong. Remember, *simply noticing* your breath is proven to activate your nervous system's relaxation response.[10] You lower your blood pressure, improve your digestion, and prime your mind to consolidate and recall information better—all by focusing on what everyone else overlooks: the breath. Tell yourself that you are enough and that observing your inhalations and exhalations or practicing your breathwork of choice is *doing enough*. Yogic breathing, along with yoga poses, is how you transform your life from the inside out.

CHAPTER 5

Warm Up

Find Your Winning Warm-Up and Get in the Zone

Do you ever feel as if you're racing around like a chicken with your head cut off? Trying to achieve the hopeless task of tackling everything on your endless to-do list? Beyond work, family, friends, community, and commitments ranging from composting to backing up your computer to the cloud, how can you still find joy in your day? Happiness feels so elusive when you're stuck in traffic. Or when you find yourself suddenly stranded with a phone at 1 percent battery and no charger. Or when you're waiting for that terrifyingly urgent call. In these high-stress moments, you're probably NOT thinking, *How can I regulate my nervous system right now?* You're probably unaware you even *have* a nervous system, or a physical body. You're totally overwhelmed. Totally in your head. And you're not alone if you feel disembodied. Most modern humans are running around wreaking havoc on their nervous systems, their heads disconnected from their bodies. Case in point: Zoom meetings!

Before the Industrial Revolution, most of us worked using our bodies, not just our brains. We plowed fields, rode horses, walked for miles to the closest market. Today, most of us sit at desks using only our heads. In one day we're exposed to more information than our great-grandparents were in their lifetimes.[1] We lead with our heads when we walk ("text neck"). We overthink everything. We have virtual relationships, texting through screens. We're cut off from our physicality. Lack of movement has disconnected us from our bodies.

My tombstone will be engraved with the words *Breath over Poses*, but as long as I am in this world, I will continue to advocate for the benefits of marrying your breathwork with a physical yoga practice. The physical yoga poses—what yogis call asana—reconnect your mind to your body, and that yoking (the literal translation of *yoga*) is what opens you up to healing, integration, and expansion.

———

Science has told us again and again that the subconscious is stored in the body.[2] You are likely moving through your life right now with habitual bracing patterns that may be so subtle, they're nearly impossible to detect. Are your shoulders up by your ears anytime you're at a family reunion? Or do you hold your breath and grind your molars when a certain sound brings back painful memories?

If you want to evolve your life, you can't intellectualize your way there. You can't think your way out of subconscious bracing patterns, especially if you don't even know they're there. As my teacher, physical therapist John Barnes, says, "You have to feel to heal!" There's only one way to discard physical or psychological patterns that don't serve you. You must discharge and release them by tapping into your body's wisdom.

Ancient yoga poses are designed to reconnect you to that body wisdom. But for yoga poses to heal your inner wounds, to propel you toward your bigger destiny, they must be fused with breathwork. Just as a match needs a striker to flame, yoga poses need your richest, fullest breath—if your goal is personal transformation. This combination—expansive breathing as you flow through postures—is the ultimate yoga magic. This pathway to healing has been proven over five thousand years. You tap deep into your body's innate intelligence, mute the unruly voices in your head, and teach your body and breath to move together in a way that nurtures you. Your body, breath, and brain act in concert, mending one another, magnifying the healing. It's resoundingly beautiful in its simplicity: The breath amplifies the healing quality of your movement, and your movement amplifies the healing quality of the breath.

Try This: Let's coordinate breath and movement. Wherever you are (seated is OK), elongate your spine from your tailbone to the crown of your head. Now inhale fully and, as you do, lift your arms up on either side of your body until your palms touch above your head. Now exhale and lower your palms at prayer till your thumbs are in front of your heart center.

Repeat. Now that you're familiar with this movement, focus on matching the length of your inhalation to the exact duration of your arms reaching up above your head. You may need to slow your arms down (I like to visualize my arms moving through molasses) so that the moment you can't inhale anymore is exactly the moment that your palms touch above your head. Exhale and slow the descent of your palms. Your hands should arrive in a prayer position at your heart in the same moment that you've exhaled all your air.

Keep going, but now imagine you're in a slow-motion movie. Remember, unlike in day-to-day life, where faster is sometimes better, in your yoga practice, slower is more profound. Attempt to do this as slowly as possible.

Bonus: If you struggle with a full, complete breath, this exercise can really help. You now have an additional cue: Your arms are an external signal of your breath speed. The slower you move your arms, the more you slow your breath, and the more relaxed you'll feel.

If you do this for several minutes, this simple breath-movement combination can unlock your primitive healing zone—a state in which your breath and body override the voices in your head. This opens up the possibility for new physical and emotional patterns to emerge. Linking breath and movement signals safety and ease to your nervous system. It turns down the volume of your pesky monkey mind. Space unfolds for your breath and body to make sweet love to one another. Your essential breath-body connection starts running the show. Harmful emotional and physical patterns—the ones that keep you stuck—start to slip away.

Why does this work? When you synchronize your breath to your own physical movements, a powerful relaxation effect occurs.[3] An internal alchemy soothes your overstimulated brain. Your focus draws inward as theta brain waves create the dreamy twilight state necessary for deep healing to occur. You enter a flow state. This flow state is the goal of your yoga ritual.

As you layer yoga poses into your ritual, it's essential to remember that the ultimate benefit of yoga—how good you feel afterward—*always* resides in how deeply you were breathing during the practice. Anchor your attention on your breath first and foremost. In complex, challenging yoga poses, this can be difficult. It's hard to train your focus on your inhalations and exhalations when you're puzzling over where your limbs should be in space and how to not topple over. I've found the best warm-up poses are the profoundly *simple* ones, because these simple poses get you breathing more deeply. And it's the rich, deep breathing that positively affects your nervous system (*not* a complex arm balance or the splits). As someone who's been hardwired to "achieve," I wasn't always a devotee of this "simple postures are better" methodology. I resisted it.

As a newbie yoga teacher, I felt my yoga sequences—even the warm-up section—needed to impress my students with bells and whistles. I'd never teach the same class twice. I spent hours creating new sequences with new poses as if they were dance routines, making each class unique and exciting. *Five-six-seven-eight!*

Many of my students liked it, yet a lot were confused. Life is already complicated enough, and the last thing they needed was to feel behind in yoga class. Where I felt the pressure to innovate, in contrast, many of my students wanted to settle into routine.

Luckily, my year of rock-bottom despair as caretaker to my dad and mom to my newborn son forced me to reevaluate my values. I hungered for that breath-body connection over complex choreography. I needed my time on the mat to soothe me. I craved time in my intuitive healing zone. I began to wonder: Could I design a way for my yoga students to experience this kind of simple yet profound yoga too? I decided to throw out my fancy ever-changing yoga sequences and focus on repeatable feel-good postures that linked breath and movement. Overnight, the energy in the studio changed. My students didn't have to focus on keeping up with a whole new sequence or learning new poses. Everyone was following along effortlessly as I repeated key movements. They were closing their eyes and going deep into their bodies. Because they repeated the same poses, their intellectual minds could unwind. They had space to glide through each movement in their bodies' own unique ways.

Best of all, I could hear my students breathing audibly for the first time. It was as if a bath bomb of calm unfurled through the class.

There's nothing more fulfilling for me, as a teacher, than to hear those deep full, complete breaths happening together in harmony, like a symphony of tranquility. How did I change my teachings to make the momentous shift happen? It was easier than you may think.

A Word About Alignment

Modern yoga has hundreds of poses, each with dozens of complex alignment rules: "Gaze over middle finger," "Sole of foot to inner thigh," "Legs five feet apart." But in ancient yogic texts, like the *Hatha Yoga Pradipika*, there are only roughly thirty to sixty postures—and most are done seated. It wasn't until the father of modern yoga, Krishnamacharya, came along that yoga poses multiplied due to the influence of martial arts and gymnastics. Then Krishnamacharya's students, like B. K. S. Iyengar, added even more postures in twentieth-century texts. The result? Today we have hundreds of rules and poses, many of which, like Warrior 1, require heel-to-heel alignment. Funny, because heel-to-heel alignment in standing lunges is *physically unattainable* if you're a woman with wider hips!

After lots of research, I realized that when it came to yoga poses, most of the original details about how they should be performed were undocumented. And the twentieth-century documentation we have was made up *by* men, *for* men. A lot of these dogmatic yoga alignment "rules" were designed to suit *only* young men's bodies.

So, spoiler alert: Perfect alignment in yoga doesn't exist. Yes, there's a way that yoga postures fit perfectly on you, and a way that they fit perfectly on me. But they're likely not the same way. Of course, for serious yogis there's value in nerding out on the specifics of how each and every yoga pose should be performed. But let's be honest: Aren't you here to get *out* of your head? And into your heart? My goal is to get you into your body, amplifying your breath, so you can access your intuitive healing zone. If we focus on what will get you there, you'll be prioritizing your authentic healing journey.

Moreover, even though "proper" alignment is often emphasized in yoga in order to prevent injury, I've found that when my students obsess about *outward* alignment, they stop listening to their *inner* alignment. Many get overly ambitious or competitive—pushing themselves too far, actually risking injury rather than preventing it.

Here's my bottom line: When in doubt, adjust every pose so you can access a longer spine. Move your feet, limbs, torso, head, and gaze—everything!—to find your longest possible spine. Stretch your spine so your tailbone and the crown of your head are pulling vertically away from one another—tailbone lengthening to the ground, top of head yearning in the opposite direction (to the sky or to the side).

Prioritizing a long spine in your yoga poses takes work, but I invite you to trust yourself. Remember those free divers from chapter 4 and let your breath be your guide. A long spine gives your diaphragm space to move in its full range of motion, unlocking your deepest breath. This is the foundation of a potent, transformational practice. Finding your longest spine and tuning in to your body through your breath is *more* likely to keep you safe and aligned than focusing on where your elbow is in relation to your wrist. You'll be connected to how you truly feel in a pose, and you'll awaken that dormant body wisdom. This is your ultimate alignment cue. Length in your spine. Ya-huh! Just this one rule. Keep it simple.

FORMULA FOR ENTERING YOUR
HEALING ZONE

Now that we understand the power of linking your breath to your movement, why simpler poses are more profound, and the key alignment principle of length in the spine, it's time to spotlight five magic warm-up poses.

The poses below are my favorites because they meet the rigorous criteria I designed for myself and my students. Over the course of a decade, I noticed that only certain poses transformed my students' breathing into an air symphony. All these poses contain three key ingredients:

- They link breath and movement.
- They do it in a simple, repeatable way.
- They amplify the body's innate respiratory intelligence.

Let me show you:

1. Link Breath and Movement

Prioritize poses that help your diaphragm move down on inhalations and back up on exhalations. The position of your torso and limbs should complement your diaphragm's journey up and down your torso. These poses are most effective since they make it easier to inhale *and* exhale deeply.

Try This: Repeat the exercise we did on page 116, where we explored linking breath and movement: Inhale, circling your arms up from your sides to touch above your head and meet at prayer. Exhale, bringing that prayer down your center line until your thumbs rest on your sternum. Repeat for a total of three to five times.

Now try the opposite breath pattern: Exhaling, reach your arms up above your head to touch at prayer, and inhale as you draw your hands down. Can you even do it? For most of us, this will feel awkward. That's because every inhale is a mini backbend for your spine, creating space for the diaphragm to move down so you can take in more air. Similarly, bringing your arms downward encourages your pelvic floor and diaphragm to float back up, aiding the process of exhalation. When you try to invert the breath in this simple exercise, you're working against your innate body intelligence. It's easier to breathe in as you raise your arms and breathe out as you lower them.

The best yoga postures complement your diaphragm's journey up and down, just as in the example above, enhancing and deepening your breath. These poses make it easier to take in more oxygen and expel more carbon dioxide—simply due to where your torso and limbs are in space.

2. Keep It Simple

Stringing dozens of complex postures together gives us too much to think about. The more you're in your thinking mind, the further you are from your healing zone—especially if you're new to yoga, and especially if you're not an athlete. Achieving true mind-body-breath synchronicity in the complex poses within a traditional yogic Sun Salutation can take years. The good news is that that's totally OK! If your goal, like mine, is to get out of your head and into your body's wisdom as fast as possible, the seated arm exercise we practiced above is *more* effective. My litmus test for the poses I teach today is that if you can't see it once and then do it with your eyes closed, it's too complex. Give yourself permission to release the yoga poses that don't meet these criteria for you.

3. Find Length in the Spine

Remember our alignment rule? Lubricating the spine is fundamental to health and well-being. The cerebrospinal fluid that runs along your spine to your brain eliminates toxins, transports neuromodulators and neurotransmitters, and ensures your nervous system works properly. So this central highway along your spinal column is of vital importance. Also, unsurprisingly, the number one reason many students flock to yoga is to relieve low-back pain. If you want to get the biggest bang for your yoga buck, pick warm-up poses that prioritize spinal movement. But not just any kind of movement. Without getting too into yoga teacher training material, some curves of your spine are naturally better at bending back, and some are naturally better at bending forward. In yoga, the aim is always balance. So we want to create stability in the parts of the spine that are hypermobile, and mobility in the sections that tend to get stiff.

To do that, I prioritize postures that take my spinal curves in the *opposite* direction of what they're naturally good at. It's like encouraging a kid who's already amazing at reading to do more math. My favorite yoga postures guide you to focus on opposing movements you might otherwise tend to neglect—for example, a little backbend in the parts of your spine that tend to round. A forward bend in the parts of the spine that tend to arch. These oppositions bring your spinal curves into a healthy balance. No surprise: Some poses promote this balance more effectively than others.

The poses I've picked below fit all three of these criteria.

YOUR WINNING WARM-UP POSES

Meet my five favorite warm-up poses, which will usher you into your primitive healing zone through synchronizing your breath and movement. This segment is the second building block of your personal ritual framework because:

1. Slow, simple movements, paired with your breath, are accessible to most bodies.

2. No matter what, if you complete these warm-ups, you'll have breathed fully, lubricated your spine, and felt shimmerings of your intuitive healing zone.

3. These movements are portable and easy to do virtually anywhere, anytime. Three of these poses can be done from a chair, and the rest require only a floor (no mat), meaning that you can do nearly half of your ritual (SIT + WARM UP) in an airplane seat, bathroom stall, or carpeted break room. How's that for adaptability?

To get to know the poses, try each for five to ten breaths. Just as we did for the breathing techniques, notice how you feel before and after. Jot down the names of any poses you especially love or that you find quickly help you deepen your breath.

Want tutorials? Download video guides for each warm-up pose at brettlarkin.com/practices.

---

1. Cat/Cow (*Chakravakasana*)

Cat/Cow is the yoga equivalent of visiting the chiropractor. When you do it correctly, this pose isolates the parts of the spine that are good at bending backward and asks them to bend forward, and vice versa. Cat/Cow is also a multitasker, opening up the chest and belly and lubricating the connective tissue (fascia) around your hips in addition to your spine. It stretches the hand, wrist, and forearm areas as well, making it especially beneficial for people who work at keyboards all day.

Pro Tip: Keep your core engaged the whole time, even as you're arching and dropping your belly toward the floor, to protect your low back.

- Come to a tabletop position (on hands and knees) on the floor. Place your wrists under your shoulders, knees over hips, ankles and toes directly behind knees.
- As you inhale, shine your heart forward, squeeze your shoulder blades together, and arch the spine toward the floor (keeping the back of your neck long). This is the swaybacked Cow.
- As you exhale, push your hands into the floor, draw your navel up and in, and make a rainbow shape with your spine toward the ceiling. Think Halloween-style scared cat. Pull your chin into your chest and look at your navel.
- Exhale all the air out of your body as you round, round, round. (It's OK to sink your booty toward your heels.)
- On your next inhalation, move back into Cow Pose and continue alternating Cat/Cow.
- Continue for ten to fifteen rounds.

Adaptations

- Sensitive knees: Place a folded blanket or cushion under the knees.
- Wrist issues: Practice on your forearms, put your forearms on top of blocks, or make fists with your hands.
- Low-back pain: Allow your booty to come way back toward your heels for a deeper low-back stretch.
- On the go: Practice in a seated position—do the same spinal movement but on a chair or seated on the floor.

2. Spinal Flex

The ancient yogis said that a person's age is determined by the flexibility of their spine. Consider this your all-purpose antiaging warm-up.

- Sit with your knees bent, one shin in front of the other on the floor, a cushion, or a long spine in a chair.
- Hold your ankles (on the floor) or knees (in a chair) with your hands.
- Inhale as you bring your chest forward between your arms. It's OK to gently lift your chin. Arch your upper back. Squeeze your shoulder blades together.
- Exhale and round the spine. Lower your chin. Round your upper back.
- Continue for five to ten rounds of breath, or as long as feels good.

3. Sufi Grind

Sufi Grind is like a shot of espresso. You stir and awaken energy in the body while you rotate your spine in all directions.

- Sit with your knees bent, one shin in front of the other on the floor, a cushion, or on the front edge of a chair, feet on the floor.
- Place your hands on your knees. Imagine your torso is a spoon stirring the stationary bowl of your pelvis.
- Inhale as you slowly move your torso to the left, then forward (allowing yourself to arch), then right.
- Exhale as you round your lower and upper back, completing this circle to the back.
- Repeat for a total of five to ten rounds of breath, then switch to the opposite direction.

Pro Tip: This also opens the hips and side body. As you circle, you may feel a juicy spot you want to stretch. Hold that position at the end of the exercise and simply breathe.

4. Sun Breath

This is a simple yet profound adaptation of yoga's classical Sun Salutation. It can be done anywhere, no mat needed. Instead of moving through all the complex postures and push-ups involved in full Sun Salutations (*Surya Namaskar*), you'll reap the same benefits by linking your breath to your movement with fewer postures. In Sun Breath, you stay standing the whole time for simplicity. As a bonus, this stretches the hamstrings and strengthens the low back as well.

Cycle through Sun Breaths anytime you want to connect with yourself or shift your energetic state. I like to do them while waiting for my tea to boil, my bathtub to fill, or my husband to scroll to our Netflix show, or as a break from work. Make it feel good for you! Speed them up or (my favorite) slow them down. Here's how to move through a cycle:

- Stand with your feet hips' width apart, arms at your sides, with a long spine. Soften behind your knees so your legs aren't locked.
- Inhale and raise your arms above your head in the shape of a big, round sun.
- Exhale, bend your knees deeply, and fold over your legs.
- Inhale, press your hands into your thighs, and come halfway up. Broaden your chest. Imagine squeezing a pencil between your shoulder blades. Try to feel a mini backbend, inviting the muscles of your low back to strengthen and your core to engage as you hold. Keep the back of your neck long.
- Exhale, bend your knees deeply, bring your chin into your chest, and return to your forward fold.

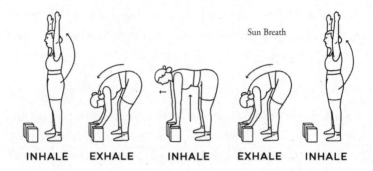

Sun Breath

INHALE   EXHALE   INHALE   EXHALE   INHALE

- Inhale to stand and circle your arms down, around, and up above your head.
- Exhale, stay standing, and return your arms to your sides— the same position you started in.
- Do this at least three times.

Adaptations

- Can't stand: Flow through these same motions seated in a chair. Exhale, fold over your thighs, inhale, and press your hands into your shins or knees for the mini backbend.
- Light-headedness: Fold forward only halfway, so your head stays in line with your seat the whole time.

5. Dog-to-Plank Flow

If you prefer to get moving quickly, this is the warm-up for you. This movement engages your core, strengthens your shoulders, and warms up your body fast! A yoga mat is preferable for this exercise, but I've also done it on carpet, on towels, and in sand.

Get into Downward Dog (Adho Mukha Svanasana)

- On all fours, curl your toes under and spread your fingers wide; see the color of your mat or floor between your fingers.

- Press down through the knuckles, especially the index finger and thumb.
- Let your head hang and move your shoulder blades away from your ears, toward your hips.
- Bend your knees deeply and press your chest toward your thighs.
- Yearn your pelvis toward where the back wall meets the ceiling.
- Knit your front ribs closed.
- Draw your booty up and back.
- Hug your abs up and in, then slowly straighten your legs. (It's totally OK if your heels don't touch the floor; rebend the knees and prioritize length in the spine.) Now you're in Downward Dog.
- Inhale and send the breath wide into your low back.
- Exhale and draw your navel to your spine.

Inhale and Rock Forward to Plank

- Move your torso forward the next time you breathe in so your shoulders stack over your wrists (scooch your feet back slightly if needed).
- Keep your hips in line with your shoulders (not sagging toward the floor). Now you're in Plank Pose.
- Engage your core to take the weight off your wrists, and press the floor away with your whole hand.
- Yearn your heels back and draw your upper chest forward to find length in the spine.
- Keep your gaze down (not forward, which could strain your neck).

Exhale and Go Back to Dog

- Draw the belly in on an exhalation and lift the hips back up into Downward Dog. Rebend the knees if needed.
- Repeat for a total of three to five times. Inhale to Plank, exhale returning to Dog.

Are You Down with Your Dog?

Downdog is home base in the vinyasa yoga tradition. You'll pause here often between performing poses on the left and right sides and between vignettes of poses to reset and recapture the breath. Why do I love the Dog? It stretches your hamstrings and lower back and opens your shoulders. Because it's a mild inversion, it can reduce blood pressure and soothe headaches. When performed with bent knees, Downdog creates space between the vertebrae in your spine, lengthening it while strengthening your upper body. Impressive for one pose!

But! If Downdog doesn't feel good for you—if it causes wrist pain or other pain, restricts your breath, or compromises your long spine—just stay in an all-fours (tabletop) position. Perform Cat/Cow as an alternative *anytime* Downdog is instructed. There's no such thing as "too much" Cat/Cow. Seriously. Otherwise, try some of these Downdog troubleshooting tips.

Adaptations

- Tight hamstrings: Bend your knees (deeply!). NO, your heels do not need to touch the floor in Downdog. In fact, bent knees are preferable and promote length in the spine. Take your feet wider apart (even as wide as the back of your mat) if that helps. Downdog is about length in the spine—find this by whatever means necessary. If possible, look in a mirror to make sure your spine is long.

- Tight shoulders: Widen your arms more (even to as wide as the front of your mat). Bend the elbows a tiny bit if you want. Experiment with your hand position on the mat. Try spinning your hands toward the side edge of the mat so the index finger points forward (instead of your middle finger). Notice if this creates more space in your shoulders.

- Wrist issues: Place a towel or blanket wedge (or fold your mat) to elevate your wrists (fingers stay on floor). Or practice Downdog on your forearms. In the exercise above, you can move from Downdog on your forearms to Forearm Plank.

ASSEMBLE YOUR RITUAL

Grab your worksheet because it's time to fill in the second section: "WARM UP (*gentle movement*)." Remember, this might be the only movement you do! Just because it's called a warm-up doesn't mean that you have to do more on a given day. A warm-up is strongly recommended if you're going to do the next segment, but we'll get to that in a minute.

For now, pick one to three warm-up exercises from the list above to add to your personal yoga ritual. Not sure which to choose? Use the quiz below. And remember: Experiment freely! On days when you feel strong, perhaps you add the Dog-to-Plank Flow to your warm-up. On days when you're struggling to get organized, or you just feel depleted, stay seated and do a slow Sufi Grind. Embrace where you are. All that matters is connecting your breath and your movement in a way that feels healing.

Quiz: Warm Up—What's Your Motivation to Move?

Not sure which to do? Love them all and can't pick? Use this quiz to discover your winning warm-up pose.

1. How often to you tend to practice?
   a. Always—I'm a go-getter and want to cross yoga off my list right away.
   b. Most of the time—Yoga is my "break" after I work on my various projects.
   c. Not very often—the day just seems to slip away.
2. What's your relationship with movement?
   a. I like to compete with others and myself. If I don't hit my step goal, I stress.
   b. I love it! Dancing, walking, even eating on the go is really my vibe.
   c. Um, it's complicated. As in it doesn't happen.
3. Without overthinking it, how would you define your day-to-day schedule?
   a. Booked solid and I'm rushing.
   b. My plans change all the time. I like to be in the flow.
   c. Consistent; I love stability and routine.
4. How would you most like to shift your energy?
   a. I want to slow down. I'm always go-go-go; I need to be soothed.
   b. I want to get grounded. I always have a million competing ideas. I need to focus.
   c. I want to get motivated. I'm always procrastinating. I need energy.
5. BTW—what was your dominant *dosha* again?
   a. *Pitta* (fire): I have a powerful ability to focus and accomplish things.
   b. *Vata* (air): I'm usually full of energy and excited to get creative!
   c. *Kapha* (earth): I'm calm, but I struggle to energize and motivate myself.

Quiz Results

If you got mostly a's, slowing down and connecting with yourself is pivotal. Perform Cat/Cow and Sufi Grind with your eyes closed. Do these movements slowly. Challenge yourself to luxuriate in each motion. If you're too wired up and need to burn off some excess energy, indulge in some Sun Breaths or the Dog-to-Plank Flow before you transition to the floor.

If you got mostly b's, it's essential to steady yourself and focus. Rhythmic, repetitive motions can help. Work with slow Cat/Cows to stay close to the earth, Sun Breaths to warm your body, and Dog-to-Plank Flow to engage your muscles and create stability.

If you got mostly c's, movement is key. Spinal Flex, Sun Breath, and Dog-to-Plank Flow all serve to create heat in the body and give you a boost of energy.

"Soulmate Pose" Checklist

I gave you my recipe for "zone"-inducing warm-up poses. If you're a seasoned yogi, you may want to integrate additional postures, beyond my list, into your personal practice. If you're not sure if a particular pose is helping you in your quest to get more embodied, filter it through my nifty checklist:

You'll know a pose is for you when...

☐ It's soothing and pleasurable.

☐ You can do it with your eyes closed.

☐ You can do it even when you're tired.

☐ You're intuitively drawn to it.

☐ You don't get sick of it.

☐ You find yourself breathing audibly when doing it.

☐ You find your breath slowing down when you perform it.

☐ It makes it easier for you to experience a full, complete breath.

☐ You feel balanced and at peace—less in your head and more in your "zone."

Use the self-knowledge you've gained in this chapter and listen closely to your body. You may notice that one of these movements, or an adaptation of it, shifts you into your "zone" faster than others. Embrace that. Follow your intuition. You'll know a pose is meant for you because it ushers you into your flow state faster than others. Through the slower breath cadence your soulmate poses help to unlock, you'll close your eyes, connect with your body, and access your innate healing potential.

YOGA HABIT: *In-Between Yoga*

Throughout your day, insert these warm-up poses into pockets of "dead time" you're not currently leveraging for your well-being. For instance, I love taking baths, and it requires time to fill the tub. I used to scurry around, trying to complete all the last-minute chores in my house while the water was running, all the while panicking about accidentally flooding my second floor. There was nothing relaxing about that. Now I keep an old yoga mat stashed by my tub and coax myself to do Cat/Cows or Sufi Grinds while listening to the tub faucet (therapeutic!). I do the same thing while waiting for the shower to get hot—I get on my mat in my bathroom. Glamorous, I know, but this is how you fit more yoga and happiness in. I'm a huge tea drinker, so while I'm waiting for the kettle to boil, instead of doom-scrolling on my phone, I perform Sun Breaths. Or sit at my kitchen table to do Spinal Flexes.

FAQ

What if my joints pop or make noise when I try these exercises?

You may hear your joints snap, crackle, or pop, just like your Rice Krispies cereal. It's OK. These noises are a normal part of life. And while the exact cause is sometimes uncertain, oftentimes it's as simple as gas bubbles in your joints getting released. Unless the noises are accompanied by sharp, shooting pain, there's no reason to be alarmed.

What if I find myself doing some other movement?

Trust your innate body wisdom. Yoga poses are meant to be adjusted to your unique body and energy. If you're in Cat/Cow and then feel a craving to circle your body, as in Sufi Grind, go for it! Sensing these physical desires means you're fully engaged and embodied, tapping into your body's wisdom. Remember: The poses were always meant to be personalized. Just be sure to maintain length in the spine and link your breath to your movement.

If I don't want to do any of these poses, can I warm up in other ways?

Totally! Although I suggest giving them a chance. Let your breath be your guide. If you're an experienced yogi who knows lots of different poses, indulge in them. My challenge for you would be to start determining which poses *most deeply* activate your breath. Stack rank them (not kidding!). This is valuable information. Perform those movements first. Short on time? Prioritize them to make even a short practice profound.

IF YOU DO ONLY ONE THING

Once each day, get out of your head and into your body by synchronizing your unique breath to your unique movement. Ideally, you'll use one of the warm-up exercises here, but if all you have time for is the seated full, complete breath with the arms up on inhalation and down through prayer on an exhalation (page 116), do that!

In the Western world we tend to overburden our intellectual minds, creating anxiety and imbalance. In order to soothe your mind and give your body and spirit the attention they deserve, prioritize yoga postures that deepen your breath and usher you into a flow state. Give your brain a break! Anytime you're uncertain about how to perform a certain pose, prioritize length in your spine. Make reconnecting with your innate body wisdom your priority, as this gives you a soaring eagle's perspective on your problems. Oh, and you'll get there faster if you close your eyes.

Now, for the rest of your life, you can lovingly look for more soulmate poses—the ones that make you literally breathe easier. Once you find them, do them every chance you get, and your day-to-day life will become even more pleasurable.

CHAPTER 6

Move

Cultivate the Opposite—On and Off the Mat

We're (finally!) about to perform what you may have originally envisioned as yoga: flowing through standing poses. This is what you see happening in yoga studios and videos across Instagram. Sure, this section is the peak of your physical exercise in yoga, but let's remember that the goal of yoga is *not* acrobatics and getting sweaty. This segment of the practice is where you become an alchemist, transforming your energetic state and bringing yourself closer into alignment with your highest, most authentic original self—the real you (your *prakriti*).

You've already seen a glimpse of this in the previous chapters. You know cultivating a connection between breath and movement is critical. You know different movements, styles, and breathing techniques draw out different energies within you. Some styles of yoga serve to energize you. Others calm you down. This can result in you feeling more balanced, authentic, and alive. Or it can result in you feeling further off-kilter. It all depends on how you're made and what energy you cultivate.

For example, my student-turned-friend Katie felt a current of excitement when she landed her first big promotion at work. The catch? Her new senior role meant speaking at her company's big event that evening. Katie often attended group yoga classes to combat stress, so to calm her pre-event jitters, she decided to practice some yoga at home before her evening soiree.

As a *vata* attracted to movement, Katie chose a thirty-minute power Vinyasa Flow video followed by breath of fire. Then, in typical *vata* style, she decided to *walk* to the event venue instead of cabbing it. Not only was she late, sweaty, and totally hyper, her public speaking nerves were still present. The yoga she had chosen to practice had wired her up, not calmed her down. This was the exact *opposite* of the result she wanted. During her presentation, Katie internally cringed as she heard herself speaking too fast, apologizing for no reason, and laughing an octave too high. Even though the event ultimately ended well, the next day, Katie texted me:

"Brett, doing yoga made me show up acting like Will Ferrell in *Elf*."

High anxiety in her new corporate role and her late arrival had definitely compounded the typical stress of public speaking. But I knew exactly what had happened on the yoga side. Like many of us, Katie had presumed that all people and all yoga poses were created equal. She'd assumed any type of yogic movement would calm her down. In actuality, Katie had immersed herself in a yoga routine that *exacerbated* her already dominant air element rather than pacifying it, which had resulted in *more* anxiety.

As someone with high air, Katie had the natural inclination to flow through poses quickly and energize herself with rapid breathwork. What might have happened if, instead, she had practiced full, complete breathing and slow introspective stretches and cultivated stillness? She likely would have felt more grounded, focused, and calm—and improved her performance. (And that full, complete breathing might have given her the insight to take a taxi to arrive on time for her talk!)

Most of us are addicted to more of what we *don't* need. We're creatures of habit. If your habit is to move fast, then moving slow seems boring. If your habit is to go slow, then moving fast sounds like a nightmare. When it comes to yoga poses and how you move through them, it's likely you'll default to what you're used to, just like Katie. It's also likely this will bring you further *out* of balance. For this reason, it's crucial to know your dominant element and the habitual tendencies that go with it. Your goal is to go in the *opposite* direction of your dominant element. Only in this way can you achieve balance in body, mind, and spirit and show up for life serene instead of stressed.

WHICH DO YOU NEED MORE: STRUCTURE OR SENSATION?

Generally speaking, there are two main ways we like to experience movement in our bodies. Some of us love to strengthen our muscles. Others of us love to feel those muscles stretching. When it comes time to perform any yoga pose, your innate tendency might be to melt into poses and prioritize sensation—feeling deeper into the stretch. Or your approach might be to prioritize structure—strengthening and stabilizing your body. Knowing where you lie along this spectrum is essential. Only then can you cultivate the *opposite* approach and design a practice that balances you. Let me give you an example from my own life.

As an ex-dancer, I openly admit that I'm a sensation junkie. My comfort zone is to stretch and indulge in big, dramatic movements. Tell me to touch my toes, and I'll fold my whole body in half. For years, I actually thought showing off my flexibility was the same thing as being "good" at yoga. I'll never forget the day I plunged my body deep into a Twisted Half Lizard. Heel on my butt, pelvis practically touching the floor, I couldn't have sunk any deeper into the lunge even if someone shoved down on my shoulders. I felt so proud!

The teacher approached me, and my first thought was: *She's going to compliment me because she must be so impressed!*

Instead, she gave me a look of concern and confusion. "Engage your inner thigh muscles," she said, kneeling down. "Hug everything up and in. You're not engaging muscularly."

Reluctantly, I backed off my full range and followed her cues. As it turned out, holding the pose in this new way she described was *really* hard. I now could feel my quad muscles fully engage. My teacher saw the difference and smiled as she explained: "You need to focus on strength, not how far you can go."

Over the next few months, instead of making my flexibility a priority, I focused on engaging my muscles in all of yoga's poses. I throttled back my range of movement, resisted the urge to touch my toes, and focused on strength. As it turned out, stretching my body to its limit wasn't helping me stretch into my best self (also, overstretching and sinking into your joints can have devastating long-term health consequences).[1] I loved showcasing my flexibility, but what serves me better is the *opposite*—cultivating strength and stability.

On the flip side, let's imagine a macho bodybuilder. For fun, let's picture a young Arnold Schwarzenegger as an extreme counterexample. Arnold might muscle his way into a Standing Forward Bend and hold it rigidly, even if it hurts and he can't breathe comfortably. If he doesn't feel his muscles forcefully contract, or experience some kind of pain, he'll assume he's doing the pose "wrong." He's hardwired to think, *Pain equals gain.* Yoga's long, seemingly languid stretches might bore him. He needs to embrace the opposite by allowing his muscles to gently stretch instead of strengthen.

It doesn't matter whether you're an ex-dancer or a bodybuilder or somewhere in between. The goal is for each of us to find the balance between effort and ease, structure and sensation, in every single pose. What YOU need to focus on to achieve that balance will be unique to you.

Cheat Sheet: Cultivate the Opposite

If you favor strengthening...

- Activate a full, complete breath anytime you feel your muscles tighten. Try not to constrict your breath or clench your teeth.
- Ditch the subconscious mantra of *No pain, no gain.* This approach sends your nervous system into a state of stress where no healing can occur.
- Resist the urge to muscle into postures. Instead, adjust your legs and arms to find more ease (this might look like bending your knees a tiny bit, using props like blocks, or coming slightly out of a pose). Don't worry about how the posture looks from the outside.

If you favor stretching...

- Use Darth Vader breath (*ujjayi*) anytime you feel yourself sinking into deep stretches. This breath generates heat and reminds you to activate your muscles.
- Imagine hugging your arm and leg muscles inward toward your bones (like shrink-wrap). Do this even if it's a "stretching" posture on the floor.
- Press your toes and heels firmly into the ground in standing poses, or flex your feet if seated. Yearn your inner thighs together in lunge-like poses such as Lizard or Warrior 2 (and if you're thinking, *I don't even know what those poses are—* you will soon!). All these techniques serve to activate the muscles of your legs.

REFRAME YOUR ASANA

Think of yoga poses (asana) as a magic mirror to cultivate the opposite of your own innate tendencies. Remember back in chapter 2 when we talked about self-awareness (*svadhyaya*) and transformation (*tapas*) through cultivating the opposite? Choosing the best poses for your practice is where those principles take center stage.

You need an immense self-awareness (*svadhyaya*) to understand your natural tendencies, and it takes willpower (*tapas*) to do the inverse of what you crave.

Practicing from this elevated awareness empowers you to cultivate balance. The result? Instead of just playing to your strengths, you leverage your yoga to evolve beyond your weaknesses. This journey toward balance ushers you toward your calmest, happiest self. The awareness with which a person cultivates the opposite is truly the measure of how advanced a practitioner is. Advancement is not about mastering more complex poses. It's about approaching the poses intelligently, choosing strategically what to practice and focus on in order to bring your unique body into balance.

YOGA HABIT: *Cultivate the Opposite*

In order to achieve a new result, both on the mat and in daily life, you have to, well, *do something different*. It starts with holding an awareness of your habitual tendencies. Then you gently nudge yourself in the *opposite* direction. If you tend to be frugal, leave a hefty tip. If you tend to run ten minutes late, challenge yourself to show up ten minutes early. This sparks the start of transformation.

If you already have a yoga practice, begin by observing how you naturally move through yoga poses. It's a great place to start noticing your tendencies, since the mat is a microcosm of your life. For example, if you push yourself too hard in yoga poses, you may push yourself too hard in life. Or if you rush in your yoga postures, you may rush in life. Next, move your awareness *off* the mat and into the world. This is your mission now: to embrace the opposite of your natural tendencies.

MOVE YOUR BODY, MOVE YOUR ENERGY

Energy isn't just some woo-woo thing. Have you ever entered a thousand-person concert and gotten goose bumps as the music started? Or felt relieved and unburdened after a good cry? Yogic science explains how life force (*prana*) moves through your body in energetic patterns called *vayus*. This can get complex, and it would take decades to understand the inner workings of how each pose affects our organs, glands, blood, guts, meridians, fascia, and ultimately mood and energy. To simplify, let's group yoga poses into broad categories, seated poses versus standing poses versus twists. The different poses have different impacts on your energy. Some increase fire (*pitta*), while others increase earth (*kapha*) or air (*vata*). Think of it this way: Some yoga poses challenge you and create more internal fire. Some postures are grounding and earthy, making you feel safe and warm. Other poses usher in more air to make you feel rejuvenated and alive.

When you're strategic about which poses you choose to practice, you can modulate the energies that are most present in your body. You can use the yoga postures themselves to pacify the elements that are most out of balance in you. I don't want you to end up like Katie in our opening story. So I'm going to challenge you to select poses for this MOVE segment of your personal ritual that serve to bring your dominant element back into balance. (Remember: When your dominant element is out of balance, it accentuates your less desirable traits and tendencies.)

Before I introduce you to the flows you'll choose for your MOVE section, let me show you how certain types of yoga poses affect your energy. Let's examine how you might further personalize them to meet your needs, depending on your dominant element. Experiencing each of these principles in your own body is the best way to understand how each yoga pose has its own energetic, "elemental" effect. Join me on your mat if you can!

Grounding Poses

Try This: Press as much of your front body into the floor as possible, right now. I'm not kidding. Lie facedown. Lightly press your forehead against the floor. If you can't do that, sit on the floor. If you have to stay in a chair, press down through the soles of your feet (this works better if you are barefoot). This is literally "grounding"—connecting as much of your body as possible with the floor, carpet, grass, sand, or pavement.

How do you feel?

My students usually tell me they feel calmer as they get their body lower, toward the earth. The more of your body that is in contact with the ground, the more that pose increases the earth element (*kapha*). Anytime you're feeling overwhelmed, anxious, or irritable, sink to the floor. This really works. When a stress wave hits me or a stupid argument starts to escalate with my spouse, I force myself to drop to the ground and lie down. Just a few moments on my back, with my body totally supported by the earth (literally *supported*!), and I start to feel psychically supported too. Grounding poses, like Corpse Pose (*Savasana*), where all your limbs are in contact with the floor, make everything feel calmer, more manageable. After his initial surprise, my spouse has learned to appreciate when I drop to the floor. By the time I stand back up, my mood has elevated too.

Nerd alert: This approach has been proven by science. Earthing (also frequently referred to as grounding) happens when your body makes contact with the earth's surface electrons, transferring the energy from the ground into the body.[2] This can happen when you walk barefoot outside. In fact, some therapists recommend it for handling stress—even in cold countries![3] Just the act of imagining my bare toes wiggling in grass or sand instantly zings carefree feelings straight into my brain. You can mimic this soothing sensation anytime you do a pose in which most of your body is in contact with the floor.

Forward folds, and any poses where your chest is moving toward your thighs and your head is below your heart (like Downdog), serve to increase the earth element (*kapha*). It makes sense, based on what we've learned about the breath: Putting your head lower than your heart is a mild inversion, slowing down your heart rate. This invites introspection, perspective, and calm.

Pop quiz! Which do you think is more grounding, a Standing Forward Fold (during which you try to touch your toes from standing upright) or a Seated Forward Fold (during which you're cross-legged on the floor and draping your torso over your thighs)?

Correct answer: A Seated Forward Fold!

Why? Because in a Seated Forward Fold, not only do you move your head below your heart, but your booty and the backs of your thighs are also in contact with the floor or ground. There is a bigger surface area grounding you, compared to just the soles of your feet if you're in a Standing Forward Fold. If you have high air or fire, a Seated Forward Fold is an ideal pose to balance your energy. If you have only a little time to practice, I'd prioritize this grounding pose.

Energizing Poses

Try This: Stand with both feet on the ground. Then lift one foot up and hold for five seconds. How do you feel?

Probably wobbly, and slightly more alert as you work to recalibrate your balance. A pose with *less* of your body in contact with the ground is a pose that promotes energy. Makes sense, right? More grounding calms you; less grounding energizes you. In the classic yoga backbend Wheel Pose (*Urdhva Dhanurasana*), only your palms and soles are in contact with the ground—a very tiny surface area. You're facing upward toward the sky. The result? Opening your chest and arching it away from the earth decreases earth (*kapha*) and increases air (*vata*), triggering a boost of energy and creativity.

Does that mean you should *never* practice backbends if you have air as your dominant element? Of course not! But if your goal is energetic equilibrium, choose a more mild backbend like Cobra Pose (*Bhujangasana*), in which you're lying prone, facedown on the floor, in total body contact with the earth, and then you peel your chest up. Experiencing a backbend from this position serves to balance you. Arching upside down with your whole body off the ground creates excess air for someone who is already air dominant.

Yogic science teaches that twists and upside-down poses (inversions) also increase air (*vata*). Twists and inversions subtly compress and decompress your organs like an internal massage. According to yogis like B. K. S. Iyengar, this "wringing" action delivers fresh blood and oxygen to your cells, improving their function.[4] Twists and inversions are ideal when you crave inspiration, fresh ideas, and (literally, in the case of a headstand) a new point of view.

Heating Poses

Try This: Do three jumping jacks. Add a burpee if you really want to impress me. Do you feel your body heating up?

Strength- and stamina-increasing movements activate your fire (*pitta*). The more movement or strength a pose requires, the more internal fire you create. All yoga poses require some muscular strength, and you should always consciously hug your muscles inward toward your bones as you practice. But certain yoga poses just require more stamina than others. These are the ones that increase fire, turning your body's thermostat up.

Awareness of your body's "heating system" and your environment is critical as you practice. Long ago, when I experimented with all the different yoga styles, I was a Bikram Yoga enthusiast. But one of the reasons I ultimately dropped hot yoga was that I could never tell how hard I was actually working. Was I sweating due to my internal heat? Through the muscular effort I was generating? Or was I just sinking into poses in my stretchy, hypermobile way *without* muscular engagement, and sweating because I was in a heated room?

You don't need external stimuli to create fire in your body. It should come from within you. Standing lunge poses, like Warrior 2 and Side Angle, increase your internal fire while also stretching and strengthening your muscles. The longer you hold them or flow among them, the more heat you create.

Cheat Sheet: Cultivate the Opposite

*If you have air (*vata*) as your dominant element . . .*

Get your whole body in contact with the floor at least once per class. Never skip Corpse Pose (*Savasana*).

- Gravitate toward poses that put more limbs in contact with the ground.
- Adapt postures to get more of your body in contact with the earth. In a Twisting Lunge, for example, choose to place the back knee on the floor, even if it's easy for you to

keep the back leg straight. With the knee in contact with the floor, you're more grounded.

- Practice at the same time each day if you can. Airy *vatas* especially need routine to stay grounded.
- Invest in some yoga sandbags. These are weighted cloth sacks that (literally!) anchor your body to the earth. Place them over your thighs in seated folds, over your shoulders in lying-down twists, and across your belly in Corpse Pose (*Savasana*).
- Practice the Grounding Flow (page 155) to cultivate introspection and get in touch with your true feelings.

*If you have fire (*pitta*) as your dominant element...*

- Incorporate Standing and Seated Forward Bends, with your head below your heart, in every single practice.
- Gravitate toward poses that have your torso and/or a full leg in contact with the ground.
- Practice heating postures like Side Angle, Warrior 2, and *Chaturanga* (pages 158, 157, and 63) in moderation. These poses are helpful for discharging your excess fire, but overindulging will take you further out of balance.
- Avoid hot yoga—you're fiery enough!
- Move super slowly. Keep telling yourself less is more, and try not to rush through poses.
- Challenge yourself to practice in silence.
- Dim the lights or practice in the dark when possible. Close your eyes.
- Practice Calming Flow (page 152) to relieve anxiety and de-stress.

If you have earth (kapha) as your dominant element...

- Incorporate balancing postures on one leg so you have less contact with the ground. Include backbends and twists in every single practice. This activates the air element (*vata*) you need to feel energized.
- Challenge yourself to adapt poses so you have fewer limbs in contact with the ground. For example, lift a hand or foot away from the earth to test your balance, even if it's not instructed.
- Indulge in heating postures like Side Angle, Warrior 2, and *Chaturanga* (pages 158, 157, and 63).
- Flow among postures rather than holding each one in stillness.
- Listen to music as you practice or to inspire you to get moving.
- Practice the Energizing Flow (page 157) to cultivate a lightness of being, a sense of being alert, inspired, and interconnected with the world at large.

FIND YOUR FLOW

If you're wondering, *How am I going to pull all this information together in a practice?*—don't worry, I've got you. Each flow I designed for the MOVE section of your personal ritual pacifies a particular element. One could become your staple. Try all three sequences, though, because I want you to have options. Every day is different, and depending on how much sleep you've had, your stress level, your hormones, and the time of day you practice, the energy you need to shift will change. It's Tuesday night and you're tired, but you volunteered at a charity event tonight for your kids' school. Take a full, complete breath and tune in to your needs. Do you need more energy? More grounding? More heat? Only you know! Check in with yourself and switch up your MOVE segment accordingly.

As always, I invite you to write the MOVE flow that best serves to balance you into the MOVE section of your personal yoga ritual. If you're feeling intimidated, don't worry; I tested each move on my can't-touch-his-toes, video-game-addicted husband. If he can do these, I promise you can too.

MOVE: "Heating and strengthening" is the third part of your personal ritual because:

1. It's essential we all move. It's rare that I meet someone who needs more time sitting. Likely your body needs more nutrient-rich, diversified movement.
2. You need to be warmed up to do most of these postures. That's why these poses come later in your practice.
3. This segment allows you to practice cultivating the opposite. The poses you choose to practice should be a physical expression of the energetic equilibrium you seek. Strategically pick postures and perform them in a way that cultivates the *opposite* of what you crave. Cultivating the opposite ON the mat then radiates to the rest of your life OFF the mat. This is how you grow and evolve toward your happiest self.

Perform each pose within your flow for five to seven breaths, longer if you like! After each pose you can do Downdog (see page 130), Cat/Cow (see page 124), or a few Sun Breaths (see page 127), or simply sit, observe your breath, and REST! Whichever of these feels nourishing for you. Always transition mindfully and pay as much attention exiting a posture as you do entering it. Take your time, experiment, and don't rush through poses. As always, your goal is to move mindfully in a way that connects you to your fullest, deepest breath.

Keep Your Breath at the Center of Your Practice

If any of the yoga poses below hurt or cause you to constrict your breath (cue NSYNC), bye-bye-bye! Don't do them! In school, you don't need to be best friends with *everybody*. Same for yoga: you don't need to love every single pose. If a pose hurts, stop. If a pose makes you want to hyperventilate into a brown paper bag, stop. You can't heal your body, mind, and spirit if you're struggling for air. Remember what we learned in chapter 4: Struggling to breathe puts your body in a state of trauma, not tranquility. Your authentic healing—your personal transformation—requires that you unite your mindful movement with your deepest breath. You can't do that if you're huffing and puffing. If you're new to yoga, move through each posture in the flow extra slowly. Sit and rest after each one. As you transition to stringing more poses together, it's critical that full, complete breaths remain the North Star of your practice. Everything else is secondary.

If you prefer video tutorials for each flow, find them at brettlarkin .com/practices.

1. Hips and Inner Thighs Flow/Calming Flow (Soothes Excess Fire)

Aura Painting *to* Lizard Pose with Clamshell Arms *to* Moving Goddess Pose *to* Triangle Pose with Arm Circles (*Trikonasana*) *to* Wide-Leg Forward Fold (*Prasarita Padottanasana*).

Aura Painting

- Begin standing, feet hips' width apart and parallel, a soft bend in the knees.
- Inhale while reaching the arms above the head, engage the core, and open across the chest.
- Exhale, bend the knees deeply, and fold forward. Let your arms sweep behind you.
- Reach the arms overhead on your next inhalation, and repeat.
- After a few repetitions, fold forward on an exhalation and step backward into Downdog (page 130).

Lizard Pose with Clamshell Arms

- From Downdog, step forward into a lunge with your right foot, your left foot all the way at the back of the mat. Shift your right foot wide, to the right edge of your mat, and lower your left knee to the ground.
- Press your left hand or fist into the mat. Reach the right arm high to the sky as you spiral and arch your chest to the ceiling as you breathe in.
- As you breathe out, return your right arm to meet your left, like a clamshell closing, and round your upper back.
- Repeat. Try to sync the arm opening and closing with the cadence of your breath.
- Return to Downdog and repeat on the other side.

- Come back to Downdog. Walk your feet to the top of your mat and slowly come to a stand.

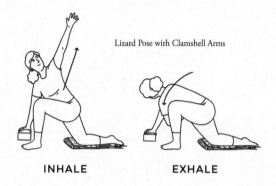

Lizard Pose with Clamshell Arms

INHALE   **EXHALE**

Moving Goddess Pose

- From standing, turn to face the long edge of your sticky mat and place your feet approximately one leg's distance apart, heels in, toes slightly out.
- Bend your knees deeply, knees over ankles, yearning your knees back toward your pinkie toes. Try to keep your spine straight.
- Inhale, reach your arms up, and straighten your legs.
- Exhale, bring your hands to prayer, and bend the knees to return to Goddess Squat.
- Repeat.

Triangle Pose with Arm Circles (Trikonasana)

- Stand with the feet one leg's distance apart front to back, your front right heel bisecting your back left arch (or whatever feels comfortable for you).
- Keeping the sides of the torso long and the chest wide, tilt toward the right leg and place the right hand on your right shin.
- Reach your top (left) arm up to the ceiling.

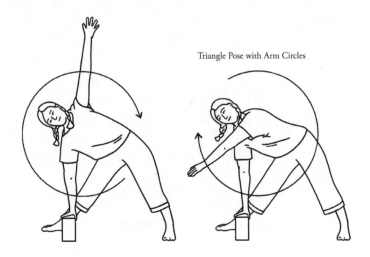

Triangle Pose with Arm Circles

- Slowly make a giant circle with this arm, so it brushes your face, moves toward the floor, and comes back to the sky.
- Reverse the direction of your arm when you feel like it.
- Do this pose on the other side, left foot in front.

Wide-Leg Forward Fold (**Prasarita Padottanasana** *)*

- Stand with feet one leg's distance apart side to side, toes facing forward and slightly in.
- Fold forward and place both hands on the ground in front of you, wherever they land. It's OK to hold the seat of a chair, a table, or two yoga blocks if the floor is too far away.
- Keep the back of the neck long. Your torso moves toward your quads.
- Draw your inner thighs energetically toward one another.
- Yearn your shoulders back and away toward the ceiling so they're not sagging down by your ears.
- Pull your abs up and in and let your low back release.

2. Low-Back Saver Flow/Grounding Flow (Decreases Excess Air)

Baby Cobra (*Bhujangasana*) *to* Child's Pose (*Balasana*) to Pyramid Pose (*Parsvottanasana*) *to* Tree Pose (*Vrikshasana*) *to* Warrior 2 (*Virabhadrasana 2*) *to* Wide-Leg Forward Fold (*Prasarita Padottanasana*).

Baby Cobra (Bhujangasana*)*

- From Downdog, rock forward to a Plank (page 129) and lower your body to the floor.
- From lying on your belly, place your palms directly under your shoulders.
- Engage your leg muscles to lift your kneecaps off the floor. Squeeze your elbows toward each other.
- Using your low-back strength (no pressing into the floor!), lift your chest into a mild backbend.
- Glide your shoulders down and back. Dip your chin to keep the back of your neck long.
- Hug your abs and front ribs up and in to support you.
- Lift your palms off the ground to test your low-back strength.
- Lift your chest on an inhalation and lower your chest on an exhalation at least three times, holding and breathing for several rounds of breath at the top each time.

Child's Pose (Balasana*)*

- From Baby Cobra, take your hips back to your heels into Child's Pose.
- Knees can be touching or as wide as the mat, whichever is most comfortable for you.
- Drape your torso over your thighs, forehead to your mat or

a block. If this is uncomfortable, place your forearms on the floor to support your upper body.

- Arms can rest alongside your body, palms cupping your heels or above your head, with the palms at prayer or with the elbows wide and the fingertips touching.
- Soften your shoulders. Take three to five deep breaths, then return to Downdog. Walk to the top of your mat.

Pyramid Pose (Parsvottanasana)

- From standing, step your left foot one leg's length back. Put your hands on your hips and now adjust your feet to hips' width apart from left to right (or wider!) so you feel stable.
- Elongate your spine as you hinge at the hips and fold over your front leg. Place your hands on the seat of a chair, a table, two yoga blocks, or your front shin.
- Inhale into a flat back and broaden your chest, coming up partway. Exhale and use your abs to fold deeper over your front leg.
- Keep lengthening your tailbone backward and drawing the crown of your head forward as you undulate up and down.
- After five to seven breaths, bring your hands back to your hips. Engage your core. With a long spine, slowly come back up to standing.
- Place your opposite foot in front and repeat.

Tree Pose (Vrikshasana)

- Standing on one leg, place the opposite foot on the ankle or anywhere along the standing leg that allows you to keep your hips level (just avoid the knee joint). It's great to have one hand on a wall or the back of a chair for support.
- Push the sole of your raised foot into your standing leg and

your standing leg into your foot. Hug everything in toward your midline.

- Gaze at a single point in front of you.
- You can keep your hands on your hips, press your palms at prayer at the heart center, or lift your arms in a wide V.
- Repeat, alternating legs.

Warrior 2 (Virabhadrasana 2)

- Take a big step back with your left foot and face the long edge of your mat. Turn your right toes and knee to face the front short edge of the mat. Angle your back left toes slightly inward.
- Bend your right knee toward 90 degrees over your right ankle. Adjust your back foot as needed for a long stance.
- Stack your shoulders and head over your hips.
- You can leave your hands on your hips, press your palms at prayer at your heart center, or reach long to the left and right.
- Hold for five to seven breaths.
- Repeat, alternating legs.

Wide-Leg Forward Fold (Prasarita Padottanasana)

- See page 154.

3. Backbend Flow/Energizing Flow (Balances Excess Earth)

Moving Baby Cobra (*Bhujangasana*) *to* Aura Painting *to* Side Angle *to* Reverse Warrior (*Parsvakonasana* Flow) *to* Tree Pose (*Vrikshasana*) *to* Dynamic Bridge (*Setu Bandha Sarvangasana*).

Moving Baby Cobra (Bhujangasana)

- From Baby Cobra (see page 155), inhale to peel your chest off the ground. Take one cycle of breath (an exhalation and an inhalation) with your chest elevated.

- Then, on your next exhalation, slowly lower yourself to the floor. Think of your spine growing longer as you breathe out.
- Repeat lifting and lowering on your breath for a total of five times. Take Child's Pose (page 155) or Downdog when finished. Then walk to the top of your mat.

Aura Painting

- See page 152.

Side Angle to Reverse Warrior (Parsvakonasana Flow)

- From Warrior 2 with the right toes pointing forward (page 157), place your right elbow on your right thigh, left arm overhead, as you breathe in with a long spine. This is Side Angle.
- As you breathe out, let your left arm lead you back in space into Reverse Warrior, placing your left hand on your left hip or thigh for support.
- Ideally, your front right knee will stay bent as you come into this gentle backbend, but feel free to straighten it if you're working on building up your strength.
- Inhale and come back to Side Angle. Exhale and flow back into Reverse Warrior.
- Repeat for a total of five times. Then perform this flow on the other side, left knee bent.

Tree Pose (Vrikshasana)

- See page 156.

Dynamic Bridge (Setu Bandha Sarvangasana)

- Move through a Sun Breath and Downdog to Plank (page 129) to lower your body to the floor. Then roll over to face the sky.
- From lying down, place your ankles under your knees. Press

your triceps, (the muscles at the back of your upper arm) into your mat, elbows bent, fingertips pointing up toward the ceiling.

- Inhale and lift your hips, pressing the feet and triceps into the floor. Dip your chin slightly to keep the back of your neck long. Draw your shoulder blades together underneath you.
- Exhale and lower your seat back to the mat, challenging yourself to move as slowly as you can.
- Repeat, moving on your breath, inhaling to lift, exhaling to lower, for a total of five to seven times.

Bonus: Abdominal Work to Add Heat (Increases Fire)

Add heat to any of the flows by adding one or both of these options:

Static Forearm Plank Hold

- From Downdog, rock forward into Plank Pose and lower yourself onto your forearms.
- Shift and wiggle your toes back so that your shoulders are directly over your elbows. Keep your shoulders and hips in one line. Draw your abs in.
- Press your heels back and urge your hips toward your chin, as if you were wearing a belt buckle that you wanted to yearn forward.
- Hold for several rounds of breath or until you feel your deep core muscles turn on. Keep lengthening your tailbone back toward your heels.

Boat Pose (Navasana)

- Seated on the ground, bend your knees and take the soles of the feet to the floor. Press down through the soles of your feet.
- Hold behind your thighs or bring your arms parallel to the floor.

- Exhale and lean your torso back in space, keeping your spine long, big toes rooted in the mat.
- Squeeze your inner thighs together.
- Draw your shoulders down and back, getting taller as you broaden across the chest.
- Pull your abdominal muscles down and back toward your spine.
- Optionally, lift your feet off the mat, shins parallel to the floor, for an additional challenge.
- Breathe here until you feel your deep core muscles turn on.

Intensify either option above by performing breath of fire (page 105) while in the pose.

ASSEMBLE YOUR RITUAL

Find your worksheet because it's time to fill in the third section: "MOVE (*heating and strengthening*)." As always, you choose what to practice for this section on a given day. Look inward. Ask yourself, *What do I have time and energy for? What's coming up next in my day? What would serve to balance me?* For example, you may find only some of the poses in a flow serve you. Or none of them do, and you skip your MOVE section completely. You might skip this segment on the first three days of your period, if you're jet-lagged, or if your teething infant is making it impossible for you to sleep well. In contrast, on days when you feel strong, you might choose to ratchet up the intensity by repeating these flows multiple times, alternating among them, or holding each pose in the flow for longer (nine to twelve breaths instead of five to seven). It's your yoga. Your life. Your body. You're in charge.

Quiz: Move—Find Your Ideal Flow

It's here in this segment that you have a profound opportunity to balance your dominant element. Select discerningly which flow you choose to practice, and change it up as often as you need to. If you're unsure or torn between two, this quiz can help point you in the direction of balance.

1. When do you tend to have the most energy?
   a. Daytime—I wake up ready to go.
   b. Nighttime—I'm a night owl! I get my best ideas when the world is asleep.
   c. I'm always tired—my energy seems to have gone on vacation.

2. If you had to describe your daily mood, what word would you choose?
   a. *Alert* or *focused*. I love getting things done.
   b. *Inspired*, *excited*, or *scattered*. I have high highs and low lows.
   c. *Stable* or *consistent*. My mood doesn't vary that much.

3. How easy is it for you to complete a project?
   a. I get things done on time.
   b. I have lots of ideas but struggle to see things through to completion.
   c. I'll finish eventually, at my own pace.

4. Which best describes your relationship with technology?
   a. I strive for Inbox Zero and back up occasionally to an external hard drive.
   b. I have a million tabs open at all times, and my photos are not backed up.
   c. I just keep scrolling.

5. How do you like to move?
   a. Fast and efficiently.
   b. Feeling into sensation and moving to the beat of my own drum.
   c. In my comfort zone, and I'm not interested in anything crazy.

Quiz Results

If you got mostly a's, choose "Calming Flow" if you want a light-intensity flow that counteracts the effects of a sedentary lifestyle (great for excess fire).

If you got mostly b's, choose "Grounding Flow" if you want a heating, strength-building flow to improve your posture and counteract back pain (great for excess air).

If you got mostly c's, choose "Energizing Flow" to open the heart, combat "text neck," and decrease shoulder and neck tension (great for excess earth).

ADAPT EVERY YOGA POSE TO BALANCE YOUR DOMINANT ELEMENT

Now that you've identified which flow serves to soothe your dominant element, you can further personalize the poses within each one (or add other poses you love). As a beginner, stay with the poses and flows outlined above for six months or more. But if you're an experienced practitioner, I want to empower you to personalize your ritual with poses beyond the scope of this book. To do so, apply the same principles you learned earlier in this chapter about what makes a pose grounding, energizing, or heating. When you put all this knowledge into practice, you create a truly personalized practice.

Let me show you what I mean. Say you love doing Twisted Lunge in your studio classes and want to incorporate it here into your at-home ritual. Adjust it to balance your dominant element.

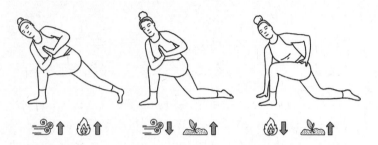

Twisted *High* Lunge with Hands at Prayer: This high-lunge variation increases air (*vata*). It's also a standing balance, creating some extra heat in the body.

Twisted *Low* Lunge with Hands at Prayer: Taking the back knee to the floor in a low lunge adds a point of contact with the earth and makes this pose more grounding, increasing the earth element. This is a good variation for someone with high air (*vata*).

Twisted Low Lunge with Hand on Floor/Hold Ear: With the knee *and* one arm to the ground, there's even more stability and contact with the earth. The other arm is now touching the body rather than muscling into the twist. This variation is ideal for ambitious, fiery *pittas*, who'd likely push themselves as far as they could go... if left to their own devices in the high lunge from the first picture.

Let's look at another example. You want to add another twisting pose to your personal practice. Which one do you choose, when remembering the aim of balancing your dominant element?

Standing Chair Pose Twist: With only the soles of feet in contact with the earth, this twisting chair posture is heating and challenging, making it an ideal choice for someone with earth as their dominant element.

Seated Twist (*Ardha Matsyendrasana*): This seated twisting

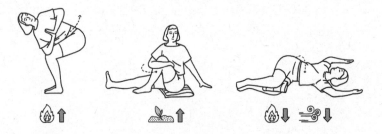

posture offers much more stability, allowing the focus to be on twisting (rather than also balancing). This would be an ideal choice for air-dominant people, who can focus on grounding down through their seat while still enjoying a twist.

Supine Twist: In this lying-down variation, the body is completely supported by the floor, making it an excellent option for fire-dominant people (to unwind) or airy *vatas* (to reground).

Do you see? No pose is off-limits when you know how to tweak it for your unique energy. You can practice everything and anything. You just *adapt* so it serves to balance your dominant element. Do *not* be intimidated. Remember, the purpose of your practice is to *balance you.* There is no "right" or "wrong." There's only your unique energy in the moment you happen to be practicing. The only rule is that you should feel supported. When in doubt, cultivate the opposite. If you believe you need to do more poses or harder poses because the other adaptations aren't enough of a "workout," catch that thought! Challenge yourself to place a knee and hand to the mat. For someone who is hypercompetitive, this is the essence of advanced yoga in action.

THIS SOUNDS HARD ... WHY DO IT?

Do some of these suggestions feel like a kick in the face? Does my advice to practice stillness and get more of your limbs in contact with the ground sound like a punishment? Or maybe you're already groaning at the idea of having to trade a lying-down twist for a standing one? I get it. This is where choosing transformation (*tapas*) comes in. The focus of your ritual is *personal transformation* and prioritizing the poses that most potently balance your energy in the least amount of time. NOT what would burn the most calories or be the most "well-rounded" full-body workout. For this, you could follow along to a sixty-minute class or read any of the hundreds of books that approach yoga as a fitness regimen. Our aim is *awareness*. You're always going to be attracted to the postures and movements that play to your dominant element's strengths. But if your goal is to cultivate balance, your personal yoga ritual works best when it reins in your dominant *dosha*'s desires. In a nutshell, do the opposite of what you crave.

This analogy might help: A tennis pro once told me I'd start winning more games once I got comfortable hitting the kinds of shots my opponents didn't like (even if I felt less confident hitting those). Up to that point, I had been hitting the types of shots I enjoyed, simply because I was good at them. But if I wanted to win, I needed to focus on what would bring me victory against an opponent, not just what felt natural.

In your personalized yoga ritual, you're playing against yourself. The goal is to step outside your comfort zone and achieve victory over internal "opponents" that cause self-sabotage, fear, anxiety, and doubt. Use your time on the mat to observe the way you tend to move through poses. It's likely the way you move through life too. Nudge yourself in the opposite direction to explore new ways of being. This is how, over time, you discover what balance feels like. From there you access the calm, radiant, authentic version of you.

I understand that this way of approaching your practice is different—and challenging. If you find yourself struggling to cultivate the opposite when you practice, use this nifty trick I developed. Indulge just for a moment in what your dominant element wants to feel or experience. For me, that's flowing movements and a juicy deep stretch. But then quickly back off and transition into what's actually good for you. For me that means putting a knee to the ground, backing off my full range of motion, and engaging my muscles. If you love creating heat in your yoga practice, embrace that and meet yourself there. Relish in a few Sun Salutations to get warm and burn off that excess energy. But then challenge yourself to transition to postures with more limbs in contact with the ground and prioritize stillness. By briefly indulging, then redirecting, you can have your cake and eat it too. Enjoy a little bit of what you crave, and then transition to what you *need* to evolve.

It may not be easy—growth rarely is! I promise: Cultivating the opposite will turn you into the most radiant version of you. A fiery *pitta*'s zone of genius is meant to glow, not combust. An airy *vata*'s is to inspire, not float away. An earthy *kapha*'s is to anchor, not sink. What's challenging for you—your advanced yoga practice—lies in the poses that serve to balance your excess elements.

FAQ

Can I skip the SIT and WARM UP sections of the sequence and just do this MOVE segment?

Unlike the other parts of your "à la carte" yoga menu, this section of your personal practice is NOT safe to practice in isolation. These standing postures require your body to be warm. If you choose not to do the WARM UP segment, please complete several Sun Breaths or Sun Salutations before performing these postures.

How much should I rotate between these flows?

As much as you'd like! Meet yourself where you are and choose what feels best for you on any given day. Each flow is best for pacifying a different *dosha*, so you'll likely benefit most from making the flow that corresponds to your dominant element your staple.

What if I have an injury?

Listen to your body. Adapting the poses to meet you where you are is key to your recovery. Check out pages 247–248 of the Yoga Adaptations Guide for detailed recommendations. Focus on what you can do. You always have the option to skip the entire MOVE section of your sequence completely if that's best for your body.

I heard I should take Child's Pose as a resting pose, but it's uncomfortable for me. What should I do?

You're not alone. In many people's bodies, Child's Pose doesn't feel good. In the video tutorials for this section (which you can find at brettlarkin.com/practices), I share adaptations that you can do instead of Child's Pose.

Can I modify or adapt these flows?

Yes, yes, and yes! That's what this book is ALL about. Check out chapter 3 and the Yoga Adaptations Guide on page 241 for support in using blocks, bolsters, and blankets and in adapting any and all practices to your specific energy. Adapt as much as you can to prioritize your fullest, richest breath, and add in your own favorite poses. Make every practice uniquely yours.

IF YOU DO ONLY ONE THING

Cultivate the opposite—both on the mat and off the mat. Recognize that what you crave isn't necessarily what you need and that doing the opposite creates the "energetic equilibrium" that turns you into the most radiant version of you. Honor your individuality. Meet yourself where you are. Choose yoga postures and adaptations that pacify your dominant element, and choose new thoughts that make your dominant element squirm. This is the work that not only balances your body but also opens you up to new possibilities for personal development and growth.

CHAPTER 7

Stretch

Embrace "Less Is More"

I was sightseeing in Japan and thought it would be a great idea to take a yoga class. Except I forgot one thing: I don't speak Japanese! I followed along the best I could. After the class, I was able to connect with the teacher, who spoke a little bit of English. She told me, "You're so great, you can do all the poses. *Except* this forward fold. Your stomach is *not* on your thighs, it's no good!" The language barrier probably made her comment seem harsher than she intended. But honestly, I walked out of that class feeling terrible about myself. I'd been practicing for close to a decade, so why couldn't I bend my body perfectly in half? As it turns out, I couldn't then, I can't now, and I never will be able to.

Many well-intentioned yoga teachers say, "Just keep stretching, you'll get there!" Meanwhile, I'm thinking, *Actually, no, I probably won't.* Most bodies are not built for contortionism—and that's *not* a bad thing! You could do yoga every day of your life and never get your knees to touch the floor when you sit on the floor cross-legged. That's your unique body. Joint variability and skeletal limitations are real.

Check this out: Your flexibility is largely influenced by the range of motion in your hips. Visualize your hip socket (your acetabulum in anatomy lingo) like a bowl. Just like the ones in your cupboard, it may be shallow, deep, or somewhere in between. The ball (called the femoral head) at the top of your thigh bone that fits into this pelvic bowl might be large and bumpy or smaller and smooth. The interplay among all these variables results in the range of motion available in your hip socket. It's not something that will ever change. This is why the Bolshoi Ballet in Russia accepts dancers based on mobility tests and X-rays. The ballet masters know that no matter how talented the ballerina, without the bone structure to enable superhuman flexibility, she'll never dance the most difficult sections of *Swan Lake*.

Some people will never get their knees to the ground or their belly to their thighs in a seated position, no matter how much they stretch. It's just the way they're built. There are 360 joints in the human body, and we experience skeletal individuation in every single one. We're all built differently.

Anatomy may seem like a limitation. But it can actually be a liberation! This knowledge empowers you to stop striving to reach the "perfect pose" someday in the future. Just as importantly, it's an opportunity to remind yourself that getting your knees to the ground or your stomach to your thighs won't summon enlightenment.

The goal of your practice is not to obsess about flexibility but to stretch into the best version of yourself. This requires introspection. Your MOVE section stokes your internal fire, increases air, and undulates the body. While you can tweak poses within your MOVE segment to be more grounding, that portion of your practice is primarily about flow. Now it's time to counterbalance by getting close to the ground, increasing the earth element, and finding stillness. Stretching in seated positions offers you the opportunity to cool down and turn inward. Yoga's brilliant sequencing serves to always keep you balanced. At a macro level, your MOVE segment emphasizes the fire and air elements. Your STRETCH segment emphasizes the earth element. So, like a ninja, you can be ready for whatever life tosses in front of you. This section of your practice also serves as a stepping stone to even deeper relaxation—Corpse Pose (*Savasana*) and meditation—up next. This segment of sitting on the floor and stretching may seem tedious or titillating, depending on your dominant element and personality. Remind yourself that this is about so much more than flexibility.

No matter how close your legs are to the ground, practicing these seated poses will help you expand your energetic capacity, release what isn't serving you, and connect more deeply with your true needs and desires. Stretching your physical body is only *one* of the reasons to practice the STRETCH portion of your sequence. The most important stretch is the one happening mentally. In this segment you increase your ability to get comfortable with discomfort, practice self-acceptance, process your emotions, and learn to set your burdens down.

INCREASE YOUR DISCOMFORT TOLERANCE

Maybe you don't love some of these seated poses. Do you hate sitting on the floor? Is being still and doing "nothing" uncomfortable? You'd rather flow, move, and get a workout? Or skip this section altogether? Excellent.

An old yoga instructor of mine once said that yoga is not just about making you feel good, it's about making you *feel*. At no time is that more true than when we stretch. Seated poses are here to give you an opportunity to practice getting comfortable with your discomfort.

Many of us feel awkward in a seated stretch. You've stopped moving and flowing. You're forced to stay still. There's not a lot going on, and you don't have your cell phone to distract you. Some sensations in your body may feel, at first, unpleasant. For most of us, stretching in stillness brings up internal resistance to the present moment.

Your mind might wander to what to cook for dinner or compose that email response in your head. You're avoiding being present to your deeper feelings. Of course, this kind of mental "buffering" isn't exclusive to the yoga mat; in daily life, many of us succumb to social media to avoid whatever emotions the present moment is holding.

Ancient yogis knew that the more you experienced this kind of slight discomfort physically, the better suited you'd be to withstand uncomfortable situations mentally throughout life. Advanced practitioners intentionally choose postures that *mentally* challenge them in order to strengthen their nervous system's capacity to handle stress. Why? Because most of us have to stretch out of our habitual tendencies to achieve what we desire. If you've already been practicing the yogic skill of choosing transformation (*tapas*), you know it's uncomfortable to cultivate the opposite. It can be scary to go against the grain of how you've always done something and approach life in a new way. This is why you have to make discomfort your friend.

Seated stretches are the ideal laboratory—a safe space—to begin to explore your edge. You don't want to get sucked into thought loops, distracting yourself and avoiding discomfort. You also don't want to go into competitive stretching mode. Your aim is to stay present and create safety while exploring new, mildly uncomfortable sensations.

Growth, Pain, and How to Know the Difference

The secret to expanding your window of tolerance lies in discriminating between "good" discomfort (growth) and "bad" discomfort (actual pain). Here's how to determine the difference:

During a prolonged seated stretch, your muscles lengthen and your fascia rehydrates. Likely you'll feel a slight quiver of effort. If that quiver feels like sharp, shooting, "Ouch!" pain, is hyperlocalized, or constricts your breath, take that as a sign to back off. However, if your sensation feels broader than a silver dollar, tingly, hot, even a bit shaky, something may be opening in a way that's beneficial. I like to call this "therapeutic sensation"—it's something you can breathe into and benefit from sitting with. You're in the midst of a transformation. If you want, you can follow the example of a friend of mine and silently chant, *Embrace the quiver* to get through it.

As your body opens and your mind tolerates the accompanying new sensations, you're expanding your comfort zone. In these magic moments, it's essential to double down on your breath. Inhale *into* wherever you're feeling sensation in the body (backs of the legs, hips, low back). Exhale, thinking *Release* and *Soften*. As long as your breathing remains full and deep, challenge yourself to stay longer with the discomfort—as long as you can! Often you'll find the sensation metamorphoses. It expands, dissolves, peaks, or tapers off. Again, anytime you feel sharp, shooting, highly localized pain, back off immediately. That's likely a skeletal limitation.

The more you practice stretching, the better your discriminative ability will become. You'll get familiar with the spectrum between "Ouch!" pain and therapeutic sensation. Over time your zone of comfort will widen. Parts of your body that were inert or numb will reawaken and regain feeling. Therapeutic sensation will ultimately evolve into pleasure. You'll begin to crave this transformative feeling. The aim is to stretch just a little *beyond* your comfort zone and lengthen right up to your edge. Just please don't go over! Your goal is to bend, not to break. Be gentle with yourself. If you can't breathe (remember those full, complete breaths?), you can't transform. The better you get at deeply breathing and tuning in to your body's wisdom, the easier it will be to increase your tolerance—in all matters.

PRACTICE SELF-ACCEPTANCE

Just as we all have a different dominant element, we also all have different capabilities—physically, emotionally, energetically. You can't change your anatomy. But you can choose to express gratitude and celebrate what your body *can* do. Chronic pain may prevent you from experiencing certain poses, but you can shift your focus to gratitude for the postures that help you. You might *never* get your belly on your thighs when you fold in a seated position. This segment becomes a place where you embrace yourself and release the desire for your body to be different. Use these seated stretches to practice loving yourself exactly as you are. Perhaps you're working with an injury and your STRETCH segment becomes where you breathe patience into your healing process. Perhaps you're ashamed of something you said, and these seated poses are where you forgive yourself. Accept yourself, whoever you are in the moment.

FEEL THE FEELS

Seated stretches offer an opportunity to increase your discomfort tolerance and accept your physical limitations. But beyond these benefits, they provide a much-needed opportunity for emotional processing. Ironically, we resist winding down because resting means we're confronted with all the emotions we don't take time to sift through in our day-to-day lives. Once you're seated, still, and breathing, an accumulation of your repressed feelings bubbles to the surface. This is a beautiful thing, but it can feel scary in the moment. Especially without context for what's happening.

Emotions don't live just in your brain. They also live in your body. As Bessel van der Kolk, author of *The Body Keeps the Score*, writes, "Trauma lodges in the body. We carry a physical imprint of our psychic wounds." Deep within the interconnective tissue of your fascia are your emotional and traumatic memories. When you stretch, these feelings can dislodge, unwind, and come loose.[1] As if they were bubbles in a champagne glass rising to the surface, you suddenly feel emotional and overwhelmed. Students often tell me a long-held stretch is making them feel angry or sad. I remind them the stretch is simply revealing the anger or sadness that already exists within them. They just weren't conscious of it. Now they are. As an instructor, I see more teary eyes in the STRETCH segment of class than any other section. (And if you've ever cried in Pigeon Pose, like me, now you know why.)

So yes, I'm telling you to put some tissues by your yoga mat. But I'm also telling you this is a *good* thing. Remember how you have to *feel* to heal? Equipped with the understanding of how emotions reside in your body, you can now leverage your STRETCH segment to let any clogging emotions from your day (or life!) surface and be released. Think of these seated stretches as a built-in time-out in which you release, instead of continuing to repress, whatever emotions you're experiencing. Do you see why floor-based stretching (which to someone across the room may look like doing nothing) can actually be an act of profound courage?

LEARN TO SURRENDER

In the depth of an emotional stretch, your job is to stay with your fullest, richest breath and then . . . well, *do nothing*. How easy is it for you to let go of control? If you're like me, it's a terrifying prospect. My comfort zone is to strive, to achieve, and to tell everyone else what to do too—because, after all, I'm *right*! As children, we often learn that if we repress our emotions instead of releasing them, we're safe. But this is an illusion. Grasping for control, shoving down your true feelings, and barking orders at others destroys opportunities for intimacy or vulnerability. If you're a control freak like me, the STRETCH section of your sequence is your very best friend (and your worst nightmare).

This segment of your personal practice is very hard, because it asks you to prioritize something our society disdains…to just *be*, instead of *do*. Witness your emotional and mental states. Don't act on them. It can be helpful to think of bowing down (often literally) as you stretch to something bigger than yourself. To relinquish control. To give up and just *feel*. To stop striving. To reprogram the voice in your head that says you should be "fixing" how you feel or doing more. Once you learn to surrender (*ishvara pranidhana*), you'll create space for new ideas and creative solutions to tiptoe into your soul.

ARE YOU A TOE-GRABBER?

For so many of us, when we sit down on our mat, the first instinct is to grab our toes and enter a stretching contest. This impulse is largely unconscious. Many of my students instinctively grab for their toes and muscle themselves into the deepest stretch. They scan the room to see how their flexibility compares to others', without even realizing they're doing it! On the mat, relentlessly reaching for your toes at best will leave you sore and tired. At worst you'll get injured by forcing yourself into a stretch by pulling with your arms, resulting in poor alignment. Ironically, this brute-force approach usually prevents you from feeling the stretch in the area of the body that's intended.

Did you know that there are more injuries in yoga due to *overstretching* than anything else? Overstretching causes your ligaments and joint capsules, which don't benefit from being stretched and can't contract back to their original size, to lengthen.[2] Lengthening your ligaments and joint capsules through overstretching forces your muscles to work *harder* in order to remain secure and stable. My advice: Back off! You want healthy flexibility, NOT extremes. Make sweet love with your breath as you calibrate your own unique therapeutic sensation. Forget what the pose looks like from the outside. Overstretching can cause physical problems. If not now, later. Close your eyes and prioritize the mental and emotional stretch that's happening within.

If You're an Overstretcher, Keep These Three Secrets in Mind

1. **Notice if you're forcing your body to reach for your toes.** The telltale sign is that your shoulders will be up by your ears and your upper back rounded. Not only have you lost length in the spine, this tenses your trapezius muscle, turns off your core, and juts your head forward, misaligning the neck. Ouch! It's a stress-inducing position—the opposite of what we're trying to achieve.

2. **Inhale deeply and find length in the spine.** Think, *Booty down, crown of head lengthening away*, elongating your spine straight like a broomstick. Place your palms face-down on the floor, on your shins, or on your thighs or ankles. Then press the floor DOWN. Pressing your booty and palms down into the ground helps you find the most length in your torso (and counteracts the urge to *reach!*).

3. **Exhale and engage your core muscles.** Pull your belly button back toward your spine as you breathe out. As you do this, either fold or twist deeper. Take your arms out of the equation and rely solely on your core. This ensures you're stretching with integrity. Respect your body's flexibility rather than using your arms to brute-force yourself into a pose.

GETTING THE MOST OUT OF YOUR STRETCH

Clearly, the STRETCH segment of your sequence has physical and emotional value. So let's get more specific about how to approach each individual posture.

Prioritize the Breath

Focus on the fullness of your breath rather than how far you've gone in your stretch. Let your breath be your compass as you navigate your body map of therapeutic sensation. Challenge yourself to breathe audibly in this section of your personal ritual. Exaggerate your full, complete breaths, like a cartoon character breathing. When you're familiar with the sound of your richest inhalations and exhalations, you're better able to course-correct if you slip into shallow breathing, or not breathing at all (holding your breath). Remember, if you can't take a relaxed, slow, easeful breath that feels pleasurable, it's not worth attempting whatever you're doing. Back off until you can breathe comfortably and laugh at your tendency to overstretch.

Close Your Eyes

Stretching is your time to turn inward. If it feels safe to do so, closing your eyes reduces mental distractions and environmental distractions, like your cell phone, an unmade bed, or even a romping pet. These distractions trap you on the surface level of your mind. Your aim is to dive below these distractions to the core feelings you need to process. Remember, if you don't fully feel your emotions, they don't magically go away. They'll surface later as self-sabotaging behavior or burst forth at a less opportune time (when you may be around other people). Yoga is about feeling more, feeling more deeply, and bringing compassion and perspective to your feelings in a safe, private space. With your body's innate wisdom at the helm, negative emotions naturally discharge themselves, are released, and lose their power. Positive emotions grow and become resilient.

Bring the Floor to You

Props and stretching adaptations aren't just for beginners. These valuable tools help you personalize your stretch and respect your unique anatomy. When used correctly, blocks, straps, and bolsters help you honor your unique skeletal limitations. If your torso doesn't touch your thighs, no problem! Put a bolster between you and your torso to achieve the same sensation. If your forehead doesn't reach the ground, bring the ground to you with a block. A circular meditation cushion (a *zafu*) or a rolled-up yoga blanket are great for seated poses, and especially great if you have tight hips and don't like sitting on the floor. Books, towels, and couch cushions are free stuff already in your home—use them to make yourself comfortable in any pose. Set yourself up for the sweetest supported stretch. Celebrate what your body can do.

STRETCHING TIPS FOR EACH *DOSHA*

You want to get the most out of each stretch, but there are pitfalls in store according to your dominant element. Even though we're on the floor and no longer flowing, the principles from your MOVE section still apply: Be mindful of your habitual tendencies, and cultivate the opposite to bring yourself into balance. Here's a cheat sheet.

If air (vata) is your dominant element...

- Seated poses are essential for you. This STRETCH section literally grounds you on the floor. You need this connection to the earth to find balance.

- Beware of overstretching! Airy *vatas* tend to be the most mobile of the three *doshas*. If you're hyperflexible, keep your core and leg muscles engaged in every seated pose. Place your palms on the floor (instead of holding your toes or ankles) and forcefully *press the ground down, away from you*. This adds even more grounding to your segment, opens the hips, and cultivates length in the spine.

- To stay focused, consider using a mantra like *Let* on the inhalation and *go* on the exhalation. This serves to anchor your attention to your body.

- Airy *vatas* often disconnect from their physicality. Encourage yourself to name the bodily sensations you're feeling. For example, "hot," "tight," "spacious," "dense."

If fire (pitta) is your dominant element…

- You're itching to either skip this wind-down segment completely or switch to competitive-stretching mode. Hold an awareness of this as you prioritize this section. You are the *dosha* who needs it the most!

- I repeat: Do not reach for your toes! Stop worrying about how you look or about getting "far enough" in your stretch. Close your eyes. Redirect your energy to your heart. Can you use this stretch as a moment to love yourself unconditionally?

- As you turn inward, ask yourself, *What would feel pleasurable right now?* Fiery *pittas* are often too hard on themselves. Let ease and pleasure be your North Star. Adjust your seated poses and integrate props accordingly.

If earth (kapha) is your dominant element...

- Calm *kaphas* often get drowsy and may slump into their seated stretches. To counteract this, find length in the spine before every stretch. Press your bottom down. Engage your core and leg muscles. Challenge your body to stay active, even though you're on the floor.

- Mix it up: Gently undulate in your stretches. Add a forward-and-back rocking motion. Think of your torso as being like an ocean wave: Lengthen the spine, coming up out of the stretch on an inhalation, and then use your core to deepen into the stretch on an exhalation. Repeat this for a total of three to five times. Once you find your magic spot for summoning stillness, soften the elbows and turn the palms upward. This invites in a lightness of being.

- Earthy *kaphas* tend to be hyperfocused on what everyone else needs. In this segment, anchor your focus on yourself. Let go of thoughts of taking care of others. Gift yourself that love, compassion, and attention. What's something kind you'd say to a loved one? As you stretch, speak these words of kindness to yourself instead.

FIND YOUR WINNING WIND-DOWN:
FIVE BELOVED POSES

YOGI WARNING: These poses are addictive. You may find yourself staying in them for eleven minutes or more (happens to me all the time). When I'm especially stressed or fatigued, this STRETCH section is my whole practice. Yes, sometimes I *only* stretch on the floor. When you have jet lag, haven't slept well, or feel the need to reset or reground, this section alone could be your entire practice.

On days when you feel strong and energized, you may be tempted to skip this section. Please don't. These seated poses replenish a depleted mind and body, reset your perspective, aid you in processing your feelings, and guide you toward transformation. The beauty and mystery of yoga: Sometimes you get the most benefit when you least expect it!

I picked these particular stretches for you for two reasons. First, their accessibility: no front splits, middle splits, or challenging hip openers here! Second, each pose stretches different muscle groups in different ways. Try each of the five poses below. As you did in the previous sections, notice how you feel before and after.

I encourage you to choose seated poses you'd rather avoid and practice cultivating the opposite, as we did in MOVE. Select poses for your sequence that stretch your tight areas. This might feel uncomfortable—and that's the point! Where you have the most restriction in your body is where you want to create more mobility. You may be thinking, *Brett, didn't you tell me there's no point? In my tight areas, I likely have skeletal limitations.* True! None of us can change our underlying anatomy, but the more you stretch the surrounding musculature, the better. Props and adaptations empower you to grow through the therapeutic sensation of stretches you'd prefer to ignore.

If it helps set the mood, you can dim the lights, light a fragrant candle, and rub an essential oil or perfume on your wrists and neck. Why not create an intimate atmosphere? A yoga mat and props are nice for many of my chosen postures, but not required—carpet or a sofa cushion can work just as well. Stay in each stretch for ten to fifteen breaths.*

---

*The one exception is the Yin-Style Seated Forward Bend (page 186), which should be practiced for a minimum of three minutes. One idea: Use the stopwatch feature on your phone.

As always, your goal is to connect with your fullest, deepest inhalations and exhalations.

Prefer video tutorials for each stretch? Download them at brettlarkin.com/practices.

---

1. Head to Knee Forward Bend (*Janu Sirsasana*)

Combining a forward fold with a gentle twist, Head to Knee Forward Bend is an antidote for depression, anxiety, and even menstrual issues.[3] It's also my go-to low-back saver. It naturally stimulates your liver and kidneys, keeping your digestive system healthy, and sends feel-good sensations through the gut-brain connection. Choose this seated stretch to open your low back and hamstrings and to gain mental clarity.

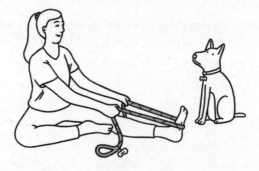

From seated:

- Begin with legs in front of you, your seat propped up on a cushion or rolled blanket if that's more comfortable. Bend your right knee, placing the sole of your right foot anywhere along your inner left thigh.

- Inhale and lengthen your spine; exhale and draw the navel in. Bend at your hips to lean forward over your left leg.
- Resist the urge to reach for your left foot. Place your hands on the floor alongside your left thigh, on your shin, or on blocks, or hold a strap that loops around the left foot.
- Inhale and yearn your chest forward to find length in the spine; exhale as you rotate and fold toward your left knee.
- To come back upright, move slowly. Use your hands to support you and walk your torso toward vertical. Breathe.
- Repeat on the other side.

2. Butterfly Stretch (*Baddha Konasana*)

Butterfly Stretch is my favorite accessible hip opener. Choose Butterfly Stretch to open your inner groin and outer hips and to indulge in a sense of surrender.

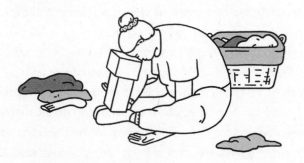

From seated:

- Bend the knees and press the soles of your feet into each other, making a diamond shape. It's OK to prop your seat up on a bolster, pillow, or cushion if that's more comfortable.

- Inhale, finding length in the spine from your seat to the crown of your head. Exhale and fold forward toward the floor. It's OK to let your torso round. Sink gently but deeply into the stretch. Relax.

Adaptations

- To deepen the intensity of this stretch, move your heels closer to your groin. To lessen the intensity, take your feet farther away from you.
- For knee pain: Place cushions or pillows under each thigh for additional support.
- For low-back pain: Place a block on top of your feet and rest your forehead on the block.

YOGA HABIT: *Lazy Yoga*

Love these stretches, but wonder how you'll realistically fit them in? You can have your Netflix and your yoga too! I love practicing seated stretches while my family watches TV. Are you getting the same nervous system and emotional benefits as practicing in total silence, alone? Noooo. But it's 100 percent better than just sitting on the couch! I have a rule in my house that if you're watching TV, you have to stretch for at least half of the show. Watching a movie or listening to a podcast or soothing music can also be helpful if you find long, silent stretches intolerable at first. The ambient noise will help you get comfortable with the discomfort of these longer seated holds. Use this as a stopgap solution as you work up to silence.

---

3. Ankle to Knee—Reclined Pigeon

Pigeon Pose is a beloved hip opener, but it can torque the knee for certain students. Reclined Pigeon—also known as Ankle to Knee—

confers the exact same benefits, but with none of the risks to your knee. By lying down on your back, you can control the intensity of the hip stretch AND keep your knee safe. Choose this hip opener to process emotions, rest, and deeply ground.

From lying down on your back:

- Place the soles of both feet on the floor.
- Cross your right ankle over your left knee. Make sure your right foot is flexed and all the way to the left of the left knee (past your left thigh, rather than *on* your left knee—your legs should look like a figure four). This may be enough of a stretch. If not, use your hands to pull your left thigh in toward your body.
- Keep your shoulders down, away from your ears, and draw them energetically together on the ground. Whether you've drawn the left thigh toward your chest or not, think of energetically pressing the right knee away from you.
- Feel your low back widen on the mat.
- Breathe into the sensation in your right hip.
- Optional: Rock subtly from left to right, like a sleepy baby.
- Repeat on the other side.

Adaptations

- If your hands can't reach behind your thigh: Place a block or folded blanket under your head or loop a strap behind your thigh.
- Press the left foot (if your right leg is bent in the figure four) into a wall. The closer you are to the wall, the more intense the stretch.

4. Seated Twist (*Ardha Matsyendrasana*)

Seated Twists gently energize and inspire you, stretching the outer hips and releasing low-back tension.

From seated with your legs straight in front of you, twisting to the right:

- Take the sole of your right foot to the outside of your left thigh.
- Your left leg can remain straight, or you can bend your left knee so that the sole of your left foot is next to your right hip.
- Breathe in and reach your arms up. Find length in the spine first, facing forward.
- Exhale and use your core strength (not your arms!) to power the twist.
- Hug your right knee inside your left elbow.
- As you breathe in, find length. Get taller, imagining space opening between each pair of vertebrae in your spine.
- As you breathe out, draw your navel in toward your spine and gently twist more deeply.
- Come back to center. Pause.
- Repeat on the other side.

Adaptations

- Elevate your hips on a block, blanket, or bolster.
- Tight hips: Keep the left leg extended long. Instead of crossing your right foot over the left thigh, keep it on the inside of your inner left thigh, with the sole of your right foot alongside your left knee.

5. Yin-Style Seated Forward Bend (*Paschimottanasana*)— Three Minutes Minimum

In traditional yogic Seated Forward Bend, I found my students unconsciously reached for their toes, tensed their shoulders, and entered competitive-stretching mode. Even when I encouraged them not to do this, their subconscious toe-touching impulses were just too great. So I just stopped teaching it! Instead, I now exclusively practice and

teach this passive Yin-Style Seated Forward Bend. It opens the myofascial back line of the body by deeply rounding the torso. It's heavenly, and
I've never looked back. The only goal in this yin posture is to succumb
to gravity. This alone is delicious and deeply healing. You don't need to
be warmed up. You don't need special props. You don't even need a yoga
mat. And you don't need to remember to do any other pose. If you stay
between seven and eleven minutes in this pose, it can be a complete
practice in and of itself. Note: This is the ideal break between meetings.

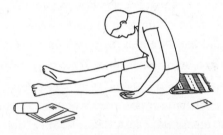

- From a seated position, extend your legs in front of you. You
  can put a blanket or pillow under your seat if you want a little
  more support. Be limp and let your legs roll out to the sides.
  There is no energy in the legs whatsoever.
- Dip your chin into your chest and round forward. Palms are
  on the floor alongside your knees, facing up. No effort should
  be expended to reach forward. Visualize yourself as a puppet.
  The celestial puppet master has just laid you down to rest.
- As you stay rounded forward, keep thinking, *Heavy head*. Yearn
  your chin toward your chest. Over the course of eight to ten
  breaths, you'll begin to feel a stretch somewhere along the neck or
  spine. Some days the stretch will be in your neck and head only.
  Others it will be in the low or midback. The longer you hold the
  pose, the more likely it is that where you feel the stretch will shift.
- Embrace complete stillness. Breathe into wherever you feel
  sensation.

If it feels as if you're not "doing" anything in this position, that's the point. You're just rounding forward. This technique uses the principle of traction to release tension in the head, neck, and shoulders. It's the ultimate exercise in discovering comfort within discomfort. Prepare to be amazed at how much taller you feel after.

YOGA HABIT: *Do Less*

My goal used to be that I couldn't go to bed unless I crossed that one last thing off my long to-do list—even if it meant I'd be exhausted and resentful. To transform by cultivating the opposite, I instituted new mantras: *This can wait. I'm doing the best I can today. This is enough.* It's no longer urgent that I film one more video, answer one more school email, or order that one kitchen utensil we've lost. Unless what I'm doing is a true life-and-death emergency, it can wait. I've done enough. When you feel the stress and anxiety telling you to push yourself past exhaustion, tell yourself instead: *This can wait. I've done enough. I AM enough. It's safe for me to do less.*

ASSEMBLE YOUR RITUAL

Think of yoga as a song, with an intro, a chorus that builds then crescendos, a bridge, and an outro. We start with SIT, warm up with breath (WARM UP), and hit a climax in our standing flow (MOVE). Then seated postures help us wind down, like our favorite jam tapering off at the end (STRETCH). Locate your worksheet and fill in your selections for this fourth section: "STRETCH (*winning wind-down*)"—I suggest one to three stretch poses for your ritual. Take the quiz I designed below to guide you. On days when you have extra time, indulge in all five!

Quiz: Stretch—What's Your Winning Wind-Down Pose?

1. How would you describe your flexibility?
   a. I'm Gumby: Superflexible, and I sit on the floor without a problem.
   b. Average: I can sit on the floor and stretch, but it's not my favorite.
   c. I'm the Tin Man: Seriously, I can barely touch my toes when standing, and my knees are high off the ground when I sit cross-legged.
2. Where do you have the most pain in your body?
   a. Lower back.
   b. Shoulders and neck.
   c. Hips.
3. What's your dominant element again?
   a. Air (*vata*).
   b. Fire (*pitta*).
   c. Earth (*kapha*).
4. On a scale of 1–10, how easy is it for you to relax?
   a. 8–10: I love to relax. Let's do a guided audio right now!
   b. 4–8: It takes me a bit, but with enough darkness and scented candles, I can usually slip into it.
   c. 1–4: Relaxation is uncomfortable for me. My mind always ends up spinning, with thoughts splintering in every direction.
5. How much sleep do you get on an average night?
   a. I'm a sound sleeper—eight to ten hours, no problem.
   b. Eh, it's hit or miss. Sometimes I sleep well, other nights not so much.
   c. Sleep, what's that? Hoot hoot! I'm a night owl.

Quiz Results

For this quiz, each question brings you a different set of answers. Based on your flexibility, tolerance level, dominant element, and ability to relax, let me recommend specific poses for you to prioritize. Sequence these into your ritual based on your goals. For example, if your goal is to increase flexibility, use the answer to question 1. If you're experiencing pain, use the answer to question 2. Looking to balance your dominant element? Prioritize the answer to question 3. If you just need to relax or improve sleep, let the results from questions 4 and 5 guide you. Remember, you know your body better than anyone. Allow this to kick off an exploration in which you tailor your stretch to your unique needs on a given day.

QUESTION 1: HOW WOULD YOU DESCRIBE YOUR FLEXIBILITY?

If you answered a, try the Yin-Style Seated Forward Bend. This will challenge you to experience a passive stretch that works with the fascia (connective tissue) rather than your muscles. Your muscles may already be limber enough!

If you answered b, try the Head to Knee Forward Bend and prop your seat up on a cushion.

If you answered c, try Ankle to Knee so you can lie down and not worry about having to sit on the floor.

QUESTION 2: WHERE DO YOU HAVE THE MOST PAIN IN YOUR BODY?

If you answered a, prioritize the Head to Knee Forward Bend and Yin-Style Seated Forward Bend. These poses open and stretch your low back.

If you answered b, prioritize the Yin-Style Seated Forward Bend to stretch the neck and the Seated Twist to open the shoulders.

If you answered c, prioritize Ankle to Knee and the Butterfly Stretch to feel into the hips.

QUESTION 3: WHAT'S YOUR DOMINANT ELEMENT AGAIN?

If you answered a or b, prioritize the Yin-Style Seated Forward Bend, the Head to Knee Forward Bend, and Ankle to Knee. These poses are grounding and help fend off competitive-stretch syndrome.

If you answered c, prioritize Seated Twist for some gentle energy.

QUESTION 4: ON A SCALE OF 1–10, HOW EASY IS IT FOR YOU TO RELAX?

If you answered a, explore the Yin-Style Seated Forward Bend for eleven minutes. You already know how to relax, and this will create a lovely challenge to deepen your relaxation response.

If you answered b, try the Seated Twist and Ankle to Knee, as these are active stretches.

If you answered c, do NOT do the Yin-Style Seated Forward Bend until it's easier for you to relax. Start with five to ten breaths in Butterfly Stretch.

QUESTION 5: HOW MUCH SLEEP DO YOU GET ON AN AVERAGE NIGHT?

If you answered a, try the Seated Twist and Ankle to Knee, as these hip-opening stretches are ideal for those who sit or sleep a lot.

If you answered b, start with five to ten breaths in Butterfly Stretch, then move into the Yin-Style Seated Forward Bend.

If you answered c, explore the Yin-Style Seated Forward Bend for eleven minutes. This will give you the sensation of deep rest your body is craving.

FAQ

Wait, did you say I can really practice just seated poses…and nothing else?

Yes. If you're extremely stressed, don't have time for your full ritual, and want to prioritize grounding, you can do just this segment. (Please remember to prioritize the breath when you do!)

Don't I need to warm up before I stretch?

Not necessarily. For a yin-style pose, like the Yin-Style Seated Forward Bend, the only goal is to let your body succumb to gravity. You don't need to be warmed up. You don't need special props. You don't even need a yoga mat. Listen to your breath and proceed mindfully.

Don't I need to do the other sections to work out or lose weight?

Surprise! Studies have shown that restorative yoga, like these seated stretches, is more effective for losing weight than vigorous cardio. This ties back to what we talked about with the nervous system.[4] Poses like the ones in this section reduce cortisol, the stress hormone. High cortisol levels cause weight gain, especially in the stomach area.[5] Seated yoga poses help you release stress, lowering cortisol levels. This segment is essential for your health. Resist the temptation to skip it.

How do I know if my range of motion is limited because of muscular stiffness or because of my skeletal structure?

Unless you live with an X-ray machine or have X-ray vision (and if you do, CALL ME so I can come over!), you probably never will. So let's keep it simple: If a stretch hurts, don't do it. If it constricts the breath, back off. Discern whether the discomfort you're experiencing feels like sharp, shooting pain or a therapeutic sensation you can breathe into. Proceed with mindful breathing. Make this whole section a practice of loving yourself exactly as you are. Reminder: It's OK to use props and adaptations forever in a pose, if necessary. They aren't training wheels—don't worry about getting "over" them. These items are here to *support* you, forever if using them feels good.

I don't like to close my eyes when I stretch. Is that OK?

Of course. You know what's best for you. For survivors of trauma or abuse, practicing in the dark or closing the eyes can be triggering. Do whatever makes you feel safe.

I've heard "emotions are stored in our hips." Is this true?

Emotions are stored in your whole body-mind complex. They are not limited to any one area. The area of the hips and pelvis corresponds to the energetic seat of the second chakra in yoga. This energy center deals specifically with desire, sexuality, and the polarity of pain and pleasure. For this reason, the hips are often associated with emotions in yoga. But these stretches will open and release emotions anywhere in your brain and body.

How long do I need to hold a stretch?

Ideally, hold each pose for at least ten to fifteen breaths. The longer the better. There's no such thing as too long. You can always work your way up to five minutes, seven minutes, then eleven. A little stretch goes a long way! And a little stretch is always better than no stretch at all. Do what you can and feel good about it.

My thoughts are spinning as I stretch. What should I do?

Draw your attention back to the present moment by focusing on your breath. Sigh out through the mouth. Tune in to your bodily sensations. Turn your attention to your breath. Tell your intellectual mind that it's safe to go offline.

YOGA HABIT: *Let It Go*

When I'm subconsciously trying to avoid difficult emotions, I find myself obsessing about anything that can serve as a distraction. Like the house remodel I want to do five years from now. I want to stay busy, strive, control, and *do* something (anything!) to distract me from feeling my true feelings. Can you relate?

Instead, in these moments, I need to slow down and notice that my desire to control has crept in. It's distracting me from some deeper fear or insecurity I need to acknowledge within myself. Anytime I start thinking I know the "right" way my husband and loved ones should load the dishwasher or buy diapers online, and I begin micromanaging, I recognize those thoughts for what they are: ALARM BELLS telling me that I need to slow down and turn inward, stat.

Rather than focusing on what someone else is doing, or not doing, or what you think they should be doing differently, I invite you to relinquish control. Direct that focused energy toward yourself and your needs. Do something nice for yourself. Soothe your controlling mind. Brew some fragrant tea, take a walk, or leave the room to take a full, complete breath with your palm on your heart. Send compassionate energy toward yourself. Stretch! Redirect your need to control others to the only thing you truly can control, yourself! Know that when you let go of controlling someone else, you receive more energy to process your own emotions and unearth your true desires. Letting go of control becomes an act of self-love.

IF YOU DO ONLY ONE THING

If you take only one thing away from this chapter, let it be this: You are perfect as you are. You are enough. Celebrate what you *can* do, and let go of the rest. In yoga stretches, as in life, less truly is more. Stretching is not a competition. The goal of stretching is to go inward and connect with yourself more deeply. Introspection is worthwhile because your emotions, your desires, your dreams matter. I beg you, please do *not* skip your wind-down! Skipping this part of your personal ritual would be like cooking a healthy gourmet meal, eating one bite, and dumping the rest in the trash. Please don't do that! These seated postures rejuvenate, soothe, increase tolerance, and promote loving self-acceptance. They're where you release and integrate your emotions instead of repressing them. This is an essential aspect of your personal ritual that will create a positive ripple effect into all areas of your life. You deserve that.

CHAPTER 8

Meditate

Solve Problems with Your Inner Wisdom

You've arrived at the pinnacle of your practice. You've anchored your energy and warmed up your body. You've moved through a personalized flow to balance your energy. And you've calmed your nervous system. All this has built up to this transforming moment: meditation! This is how you access your deepest wisdom, grace, and compassion—your happiness.

The proven power of meditation has been affirmed over millennia. Today it's acknowledged by sophisticated (and once-skeptical) medical science. Yet even now, it's glossed over—or even skipped entirely—in many modern Western yoga classes. How ironic! The physical postures were created for one simple reason: to prepare you for meditation. The underlying reason yogis performed yoga poses was to prepare the body to sit *still*! (Counterintuitive, right?) They noticed they could meditate for longer if they performed physical postures first.

A kindergarten teacher in my neighborhood uses this same technique. Every morning she asks her five-year-old students to do "the wiggles," shaking and stretching their bodies, before asking them to sit still at their desks to stretch their brains. This is common sense.

Get the physical fidgets out of the way, and then you can clear the mental fidgets. It's much easier to observe the unwieldy mind after you've burned off some kinetic energy, as we do in the MOVE section. This is what we've been preparing for all along.

ARE YOU WILLING TO WITNESS YOUR MIND?

"I tried to meditate once—all I got was pins and needles in my legs."

"My mind just kept spinning—so I quit."

"It's impossible for me to think of nothing."

I hear variations of these complaints ad nauseam. Perhaps you too have bought into the meditation myth, the misconception that meditation means emptying your mind. This could not be further from the truth. Meditation is the practice of *observing* your mind, and it takes a willingness to witness the inner stories you're telling yourself. To listen to the never-ending chatter. To observe negative thought patterns in your head as if they were clouds drifting across the sky. And to do so without judgment.

Over time, your meditation might result in a connection to an expansive sense of peace. A realm beyond your mind. Your mind's chatter slowly fades, and you ascend into effortless quiet and calm. But when you're first starting out, this sensation can be rare. I promise, as you practice, you'll access this inner wisdom more quickly and more often. But new meditators often get stuck in this trap: They begin to judge themselves and their process. They think, *I'm not doing it right* because instead of witnessing a white light or experiencing nirvana, they're *overwhelmed* by the frantic pace of their own mind. It's not you!

Human beings have a lot of thoughts. In fact, ancient yogis believed that you have one thousand thoughts in the time it takes to blink your eyes. A few of these thoughts percolate to the surface of your consciousness. All the rest sink into the murk of your subconscious. What's fascinating is that regardless of whether these thoughts become conscious or stay in the subconscious, they remain with us, taking up valuable storage space in our minds and souls. Remember how author Bessel van der Kolk discovered that the body keeps score—literally? If you don't move your body, whatever is trapped in your subconscious doesn't move either. If you don't train your mind through meditation, negative thoughts can cloud and clog your precious headspace forever.

If you've ever been overwhelmed by your own mind when you close your eyes, consider this: The yogic idea of a thousand thoughts per blink originated thousands of years ago. Today it's probably more like one hundred thousand thoughts per blink!

Thanks to the ubiquity of the internet, Netflix, multitasking on our various devices, and porous boundaries between work, family, friends, and the self, we're inundated with more facts and feelings than ever before. In a chain reaction, each new piece of information triggers more thoughts, more ideas, more emotion, more mental clutter. The best smartphone in the world has limited storage, and even supercomputers break down unless you pause, audit the files, and empty the virtual trash. Your body and mind are no different. You need time to categorize, sort, store, file, and process information.

A colleague once bemoaned to me that his laptop home screen was always cluttered. He'd sit down to do work, see the home screen, and immediately feel defeated. He called it "the home screen from hell." Yet he could never find the time to organize his files and delete the ones he didn't need.

To me this is a profound metaphor. If you choose *not* to meditate, you're accepting the home screen from hell as your mental default. You're always overwhelmed and can't recall information you need when you need it. Your operating system is bogged down. You choose to accept a life of permanent disarray and discouragement, cluttered with outdated programming from your childhood, as well as insidious "malware" you've picked up on your life's journey. Yikes! Unless you make the choice—and make the time—to occasionally declutter your mental home screen, this sense of chaos overwhelms and undermines your entire life. The result? Stress, self-sabotage, or undesirable health conditions.

Observing your thoughts—good, bad, or indifferent—has immense value. For most of us, meditation is the *only* opportunity to witness our overactive minds from a place of calm. Eons ago, humans had more time to be alone with their thoughts. People took long meditative journeys on foot or horseback to get food and water. They made spiritual pilgrimages. They rested in silence by a fire each night. They gazed up at the stars.

In this unstructured time, the brain repaired itself. We deleted thought-files we no longer needed and emptied the metaphorical trash. Long ago, life provided us with more pockets of time to orient our attention inward and find calm.

Today, instead of turning inward to feel more deeply, we turn outward. We numb ourselves with distractions instead of connecting with our authentic selves. We anesthetize ourselves in front of Netflix. We listen to a podcast while playing *Candy Crush* in a grocery store line, amid the Muzak and chatter in the background. Our evenings are literally spent with a small supercomputer phone in one hand while a TV or video game blares. The pings and beeps of notifications popping up every two seconds keep a steady stream of new information flowing—spawning more thoughts, more mental reactivity. Most of this content is pure distraction. It doesn't serve to make us happy. It doesn't help us pursue our purpose. Quite the contrary!

Try This: Start a stopwatch on your phone so you can time yourself. Now close your eyes, sit back, and observe what you're thinking about. Categorize each thought as it comes up:

- Worry
- To-Do List Item
- New Idea
- Question

I visualize slotting each of my thoughts into a file folder with the corresponding heading. This labeling technique helps me achieve distance from my thoughts. It opens up space to process how I *really feel* beneath the mind's chatter. For most of my students, practicing this labeling and distancing can be uncomfortable. How long are you able to do this before you feel your hand twitch and you capitulate and reach for your phone? Thirty seconds? Two minutes? Three?

Isn't it interesting? The pull toward a device or distraction is almost irresistible. We've all been wired to prioritize taking in *new* information: scrolling the news, reading a friend's text, refreshing our Instagram feeds. Content providers intentionally design their products to be neurologically addictive.[1] What happens if you never take a break from this ever-burgeoning information overload? Your thoughts run amok in a state of cognitive overwhelm, resulting in anxiety, stress, and burnout.

Meditation challenges you to choose a different path. Instead of reaching *outward* for what's *new*, reach *inside* to find what's *true*. Ask yourself: *How do I feel? What do I really want and need?*

Better still, by observing your thoughts through meditation, you can actually *elevate* those thoughts. Many of the most successful people in our society, from professional athletes to corporate titans to Madonna, make time to meditate. Why? To clear their minds and focus on what matters most. The challenge? Some of your internal programs can be hard to face. You may squirm at these thought patterns. This is where meditation becomes a practice of tolerance and nonjudgment. Can you increase your ability to stay present, and witness the programs running your life, without judging yourself?

TRANSCENDING A POLARIZED WORLD

This may not be true on other planets, but our planet is governed by the energetic principle of polarity. It's not just the sciences of electricity, magnetism, and electronic signaling that are based on polar-opposite charges. Polar opposites are everywhere: day and night, hot and cold, wet and dry, love and hate. You see this in the opening of the Bible ("God separated the light from the darkness"), the yin/yang symbol from ancient China, and mythologies from around the world (full of tales of good versus evil). Being and doing are polar opposites. So are thinking and feeling. The list goes on and on.

Over 250 million years, our brains have continuously evolved to navigate life on earth. But the oldest part of our brain, our reptilian brain, governs our most primitive instincts of survival: those involving fear, hunger, and procreation. This primitive brain perceives only a world of polarity: *Is it safe or unsafe? Am I happy or sad? Is this information true or false? Is this person friend or foe? Villain or hero?*

This binary thinking may have saved our species. And of course there are shades of gray, the world that exists in between yes and no. But let me plant a big caution sign here, because while we DO have the ability to perceive shades of gray, the *primary* impulse of our instinctive reptilian brain—*first and foremost*—is to perceive polarity.[2] Let me give you an example.

Ever notice that you're quick to jump to worst-case conclusions, to catastrophize? For most of us, the mind initially leaps to the worst possible scenario; your boss asking, "Can you swing by my office?" in your head becomes *I'm going to get fired.*

High-contrast information is thrilling to our primitive reptilian brain. Polarity is why tabloid news and social media are so tantalizing. They heighten the extremes. In the news lineup, if it bleeds, it leads. Splashy stories trigger our immediate response. They bypass our rational brains and go straight to the most primitive part of our minds—the part that is reactive, fearful, or excited and that is linked to our neurological stress response.

In order to upgrade our human operating systems, we must stop this either/or thinking from running our lives when we're stressed (causing even more anxiety). Practicing meditation strengthens the most evolved, higher centers of your brain: the prefrontal cortex and the pituitary gland, which secretes the peptides and hormones that fuel your current mood.[3] This master gland is symbolically represented by the red dot (*bindi*) between the eyebrows, the space yogis refer to as "the third eye." If this all sounds far-fetched, there are thousands of neuroscience textbooks and peer-reviewed articles in medical journals that back up the power of this master gland. Bottom line: Meditation doesn't just elevate your thinking, it helps you leverage the most powerful parts of your beautiful brain.

EVERYTHING YOU NEED IS WITHIN YOU

If I asked, how would you describe yourself? Who are you? You might tell me you're a Capricorn, a mom, a sister, a dreamer, an artist, a procrastinator, an accountant, or a dog lover. You might tell me you love pizza but hate pickled onions. What if I said none of this is really true? Or really you? What if you're describing the *least* of you—your *small self*? Beyond your intellectual identity, your cultural labels, talents, likes, and dislikes, you have within you an expansive and profound identity—a *big self*. It's deep within you, so deep that it may have gotten buried or lost. While part of you adores black cats, feels strongly about human rights, and loathes cheesecake, the *best you* is elevated in a perpetual state of compassion, calm, and happiness. Ancient yogis had a philosophy to explain these two identities that coexist within us.

> **Universal Consciousness (Brahman):** The yet-to-be-thought-of wisdom residing in cosmic intelligence. The raw data of the universe where polarity dissolves. Deep, limitless love. Picture the ocean.
>
> **Your Unique Spirit (Atman):** Universal Consciousness (see above), but with your individuality—your unique identity—attached. Picture a droplet of water.

The idea is that each of us is a reflection of the divine genius of the universe. You, I, and God/Universal Consciousness, we're all made up of the same ingredients. Imagine your unique spirit (Atman) as the droplet, finite, separate, and structured. Unlike the formless ocean, the droplet has individualization attached. It's identical to the ocean, except for the fact that it has a finite shape. That singularity creates your separate and unique soul, resulting in your special talents and preferences as a physical being. You are the individual drop of water, AND you are also the ocean. Just as every snowflake is unique, each snowflake is also snow. You are separate, AND you are part of something much greater. This brings up the question, Which part of you do you want to connect with? The part of you that is singular and opinionated and has form? Or the part of you that is expansive, calm, and infinite?

The problem, according to yogic philosophy, is that most of us believe we *are* our individuality. We live in the misconception that our personality and thought loops are the sum total of our identity. We've somehow lost the knowledge that in addition to being unique souls, we are made of the same stuff as the universe. As much as you are *you*, you are also Universal Consciousness, calm and at peace. You are divine intelligence walking around planet Earth—with a cute personality costume on.

You're already familiar with the part of you that makes up your individuality: you know you like the forks organized by size, hate washing your clothes with bleach, and prefer the window seat over the aisle when you travel. Why not dedicate a little time each day getting to know that part of you that is pure universal acceptance and love? The part of you that is present, radically open, crazy compassionate, and connected to a profound creative source?

Meditation helps you remember that you are not your day-to-day worries and thoughts. Who you are is so much bigger than your to-do list. Your unique body/mind, your *prakriti*, which we learned about earlier, houses your soul during your time here on earth. Meditation is your chance to purposefully channel this infinite, blissed-out aspect of your identity. It serves as a gateway for your individual soul—Atman—to remember that while it's unique, it's also part of a universal whole, Brahman. This exposes you to the loving, solution-filled version of yourself that's intrinsically connected to everyone and everything: your highest self. The real you.

> **Your highest self:** Your unique individual consciousness (Atman), remembering its true identity as cosmic, divine intelligence (Brahman) and acting in the world accordingly.

Meditation cultivates this relationship with your highest self. And it's not just calm relaxation. In meditation, you access new, unprocessed thoughts and fresh ideas from the cosmos. My dear friend and yoga teaching partner, seventy-five-year-old Guru Singh, has been meditating for more than fifty-five years. He describes meditation as a place where you can access the "raw intelligence of the universe." Instead of using our binary, reptile way of thinking, rooted in earthly polarity, through meditation you can *evolve*. You can connect with a higher plane of consciousness and inspiration. In meditation you observe without judgment your habitual thinking, focus on your breath, and draw your awareness up your spinal column, through the crown of the head, transcending to something greater. Here, high above your day-to-day thoughts, you stay open, present, curious, and calm…and simply *wait*. With practice you become so relaxed that you can tap into a network of new ideas.

Guru Singh describes these insights as "raw intelligence" because it can feel a bit like accessing the alphabet before those letters become familiar words. Instead of the same old ideas, you sense into something new. In this headspace, you can rewire the kind of negative, either/or thinking that's so prevalent on this plane of consciousness. You channel fresh ideas from the cosmos instead. Thanks to meditation, you can enter a higher and happier consciousness. A place where your worn-out stories and troubling narratives dissipate into simpler elements, then reshape and re-form themselves in new ways, into more compassionate stories.

Ultimately, though, your goal isn't just to access the "raw intelligence" Guru Singh describes. You want to bring your nuanced perceptions, your calm, and your creative solutions back down to earth and embody them in this world.

Yogic philosophy states that the divine brilliance of the universe lives within YOU. Meaning you already know the answers you seek. I used to think that the more I learned intellectually—the more I reached outward—the more fulfilled I'd become. Turns out the opposite is true. The more I create time and space to go inward through meditation and the more I connect with ingenious, unique solutions that would never occur to anyone but me, the happier I am.

OPEN UP TO EUREKA MOMENTS

Ever had a brilliant idea pop into your head while taking a shower? You're shampooing your hair thinking some issue has to be *this* way or *that* way. You're stuck in a binary, polarizing thought loop. Suddenly, *whoosh!* A creative solution hits you. Polarity dissolves. You receive a bolt of insight, like a gift from heaven above. Or maybe this has happened to you during your daily run, or while you were driving, or knitting.

Typically, these eureka moments can't be summoned—they just occur by chance, and all too rarely. That is precisely what makes meditation the crown jewel of your yoga tool kit: It enables wisdom, insight, clarity, and creativity to flow through you. Instead of hunting down a solution, you become radically present. In doing so you open yourself up to *receive* your own innate wisdom. In meditation is where I channel my best ideas. You might come to your meditation yearning for clarity about a particular problem, but I find I get the best answers when I let the specifics go. I find that asking myself a particular question while I'm meditating brings my intellectual mind back online. And the intellect is exactly what I'm working to transcend. Bring openness and curiosity to your practice. The universe knows what to route through you, if you make yourself available.

Healers, innovators, and seekers—millennia ago as well as today—prioritize making time for meditation. This is your chance to cultivate eureka moments! Once my students understand how developing this skill can solve their real-world problems, even my most reluctant meditators become avid about developing a practice. Instead of constantly reaching outward to triage your woes—googling for advice, phoning a friend, polling your family—sit in meditation and turn inward.

In just a minute, you'll learn a three-step meditation technique to connect you with your highest and happiest self (and on page 218 you'll find some adaptations that will support you). Before this magical adventure, though, let's get practical—your best meditation experience can't happen if you're uncomfortable on the floor and your foot's asleep. How are you supposed to sit?

HOW TO SIT FOR MEDITATION

Myth-buster moment! You aren't automatically disqualified from meditation if you can't sit on the floor with perfect posture. Sitting upright with an erect spine for long periods is a skill that may take years to master. Yoga poses weren't designed only to alchemize your energy, but also to strengthen and stretch the parts of your body that support you sitting still in meditation. Without training and practice, *no one* can sit cross-legged on the floor for long. Moreover, depending on your unique hip structure (discussed in chapter 7), sitting comfortably cross-legged on the ground may *never* be viable. Luckily, you have options:

On a Chair

- Scooch toward the front edge of your chair to find a long spine: shoulders over hips, ears over shoulders. You should feel your abs and low back working to keep your spine erect.
- Ensure your feet are on the floor, directly under your knees. Ideally, your knees are at a right angle. If you're petite, place yoga blocks or books underneath your feet to ensure that the full sole of your foot is grounded.
- If this position feels too challenging to hold for several minutes, or your back starts to ache, place a pillow behind your lower spine for support.

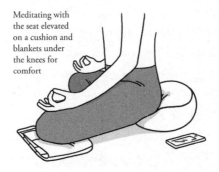

Meditating with
the seat elevated
on a cushion and
blankets under
the knees for
comfort

On a Cushion

After years of meditating cross-legged on the floor, these days I *always* meditate on a cushion for extra comfort. While a fancy yoga cushion (*zafu*) can be nice, a pillow or couch cushion works equally well, and costs nothing. Whatever cushion you choose, make sure that it props you up so your hips are higher than your knees. This prevents your feet from falling asleep. Also, please never feel pressured to sit in Lotus Pose (shins crossed, heels resting on the tops of your upper thighs). This torques the knee, so I choose not to do it. You don't need to either.

- Sit on the front edge of the cushion (this supports your low-back curve and sets your spine up for optimal alignment).
- Stack your shoulders over your hips, your ears over your shoulders.
- Cross your legs in front of you with both feet on the floor, one heel in front of the other. Place a rolled or folded blanket under your knees or ankles for additional support.
- Rest your hands, palms faceup, high on your thighs—near your hips—so your shoulders can draw back and your heart can lift. Placing the backs of your hands directly on top of your knees causes many people to lean forward or round the upper back, throwing off the ideal alignment of the spine.

- Use a wall! Sitting in this position, even with a cushion, is *work* for your abdominal and erector spinae muscle groups. While you're building strength, have your back against the wall and lean into it for support if you get tired.

In Hero's Pose (*Virasana*)

This position is ideal if you have tight hips.

- Place a blanket on the floor for extra knee padding.
- Sit on your shins, placing your seat on a yoga block, cushion, or stack of books between your heels.
- Optional: Add a yoga bolster or additional folded blanket between your calves and seat.

Each of these positions requires core and low-back strength, which you'll build over time. To work your way up, you could sit and meditate for three minutes, then return to Corpse Pose (*Savasana*). Make meditation *pleasurable* for you. Be patient and practice self-compassion as your body gets used to sitting still with a long spine.

Corpse Pose (Savasana)

If none of these poses work for you, meditate lying down in Corpse Pose (*Savasana*). Though the name sounds unpleasant, it's supposed to convey that both the body and the mind are at rest. Your comfort is essential. If your back aches or your foot is asleep, this discomfort will consume you. It takes remarkable self-control to get beyond the annoyance, and in the meantime you're erasing the opportunity to observe your thoughts. Savasana is a full-body release. You're completely supported by the floor. This allows you to enter a deep state of rest. If observing your thoughts from this position works for your meditation, meditate here! But be aware of the risks... namely, that your meditation might quickly morph into a nap. Beyond a potential meditation position, Corpse Pose is a yoga pose in its own right. In fact, many yogis consider it the most important pose to practice in a sequence. It's where you stop to pause and soak in all the benefits of the poses that came before. It's your chance to practice *being* instead of *doing*. So don't miss out.

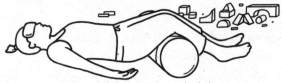

Savasana with an eye pillow and bolster under the knees

To Take *Savasana*

From seated

- Place a bolster or pillow under your knees. This will allow your low back to widen and relax once you're fully lying down on the ground.
- Press the soles of your feet into the floor. Hold the backs of your thighs and lift your heart. Now, drawing the navel back, roll down to lie on the floor one vertebra at a time (a fun last moment of core work!). Your back and the back of your head now are flat on the mat.
- Press the soles of your feet into the floor again, lift your hips and low back up off the mat, and lengthen your tailbone toward your heels. This should feel like a mini pelvic thrust. Lower your bottom back down to the mat, and notice if you feel more length in your lower spine.

- Press your elbows into the floor and draw your shoulder blades toward one another. This gently opens the chest.
- Lengthen one leg, then the other, over the bolster or pillow you already have in place.
- Put your left hand to your heart and your right hand to your belly. Or let each arm extend along either side of your torso. Choose whichever is most comfortable for you.
- Visualize the bones of your body getting heavy, weighing down the mat. Let the floor fully support you, with no effort on your part.
- Let go of any effort to shape or control the breath.
- Stay here for as long as you can: two to five minutes to end your personal ritual, or, if you have time for an extended practice, ten minutes or more.

Fun fact: You don't have to choose between Corpse Pose and meditation. A true yogi does BOTH. You can do this after meditation, making it the very last element of your ritual. Or you can transition from your STRETCH section to Corpse Pose, then exit to come into a meditation seat. I personally like to do *Savasana* first, before I meditate. Here's exactly how to exit Corpse Pose to either come into a meditative seat or close your practice.

To Exit *Savasana*

- Bend your knees, place the soles of your feet on the bolster or pillow that was under your knees, and roll to your right side. Rest here for a moment.
- Use your left arm to press your body up away from the floor. Keep your head heavy, eyes closed, until you reach a seated cross-legged position.

- Inhale, take your arms out to your sides horizontally, then move them up so your palms touch above your head.
- Exhale, drawing your hands at prayer down the centerline of your body. Close your practice here, or, if you haven't meditated yet...
- Take the appropriate hand position (*mudra*) for the version of the ball of light visualization you plan to practice (see page 214). Sit up on a cushion or find your comfortable seat. Begin the meditation below.

No matter which posture you choose to meditate in, prioritize keeping length in your spine. Sitting upright with your shoulders over your hips and your ears over your shoulders allows for your fullest, richest breath. Again, it's your breath that fuels your transformation and becomes the vehicle for your meditative journey.

HOW TO MEDITATE IN THREE STEPS

Thousands of guided meditations exist on the internet. I alone have more than a hundred on my YouTube channel, each with a specific theme and purpose. However, almost all follow the same fundamental structure I present here. If your goal is to overcome either/or thinking, tap into your unique genius, and channel creative wisdom to improve your life and relationships, this three-step framework works the best: witness, connect, reground. The way we'll personalize this segment of your ritual is a little different from what we did with the others. Everyone is going to use this same three-step meditation as their base. Then, after we've outlined each step, I'll offer you some variations on the second portion of it (*connect*) to best soothe your dominant element.

Step 1: *Witness* the Stories You're Telling Yourself

Just as your diaphragm is a muscle powering your breathing, there's a muscle of awareness that's powering your choices. Just as every attempt to observe your breathing counts, so does every attempt to compassionately notice your inner dialogue. Once you're in your comfortable meditation seat, close your eyes and draw your attention inward. Likely, there's a lot going on in your brain. Here's how to elevate and gain awareness of your thoughts:

- **Pause.** Notice how you're breathing right now. Invite in a full, complete breath.
- **Listen to the stories currently playing inside your head.** Imagine you tuned in to a radio station in your car midsong. Really listen to it and spend time noticing what that "song" is. Don't change the station, dismiss the song, or try to stop it. Let each thought unfurl, as if it had nothing to do with you. You're just watching.
- **Strive to notice all this inner dialogue without judgment.** If it helps, try on the labeling exercise from page 200 to categorize your thoughts. Alternately, visualize yourself as the sky and your mental chatter as drifting clouds. Allow yourself to watch your thoughts change as they float beyond sight.
- **Send yourself nourishment and compassion as you witness your mental chatter.** Your awareness of these thoughts is *without judgment.* Remind yourself that you're just an observer right now. Think, *I am* not *the voices in my head.*

Note: If your inner dialogue becomes overwhelmingly nasty or cruel, shift your attention to your breath. Stop observing your thoughts. Instead, strive to connect with your physical sensations.

Place your hands palms-down on your thighs or chest. Touching your own body soothes the nervous system and draws you back into the present moment. If emotions come up and you feel your eyes welling with tears, don't fight them. Often we feel better after a good cry. You can also open your eyes and take a break.

Step 2: *Connect* with Your Divine Self

Tapping into the real you—that calm, compassionate inner wisdom—can be challenging. I've found the power of visualization immensely helpful. My favorite technique comes from Alan Finger, the founder of ISHTA yoga, who learned it from his father, a student of Yogananda, the famous yogi from *Autobiography of a Yogi*. I love the ball of light visualization because it clears away psychic debris and opens an energetic pathway up and down the spine. Ancient yogis viewed the spinal cord as the meridian channel (*nadi*) that connects you to your divine cosmic intelligence and bliss.

Ball of Light Visualization

- After observing your thoughts without judgment, shift your attention to the length of your spine. Visualize your seat rooting down and the crown of your head lifting up.
- As you inhale, silently think the sound *hum*. Visualize a ball of light rising from your tailbone to the space between your eyebrows.
- As you exhale, mentally think the sound *sa*. Visualize the ball of light descending from your midbrain down to the base of your spine, like an elevator moving down.
- Repeat. Keep thinking *hum* (ball of light moves up the spine), *sa* (ball of light moves down the spine). Link the ascent and descent of this light with the cadence of your unique breath. *Hum sa* translates to "I am that." In yogic philosophy, it means identifying oneself (a water drop) with the universe (the ocean).

- After ten to twelve rounds, allow the ball of light to stay elevated in your midbrain. Think *hum* as the ball of light glows in the center of the brain. Think *sa* as you expand the ball of light so it radiates in all directions (up, down, forward, back, and from side to side). Sense your mind blossoming into an elevated field of awareness.

Step 3: The Profound *Reground*

Unless you're a full-time monk, transcending your body to exist fulltime in an otherworldly state of spiritual bliss isn't that useful. Your aim is more practical—and achievable: to live and act as your happiest self in your own unique life in *this* world. To do this you have to do something called regrounding to channel any energetic wisdom you've accessed at the end of step 2 back down into your daily life.

Sadly, most meditation techniques fail to reanchor us. (If you've ever felt dizzy, spacey, or headachy after meditation, this is likely why.) The goal in regrounding is to siphon the subtler energies you've experienced in your meditation *down* through your physical body so you can act on them as you move through *this* world. Here are three of my favorite regrounding techniques for you to try out.

1. **Palm rubbing.** Press your hands into prayer at the heart center, then rub your palms vigorously together for a full minute. Creating heat and friction between your palms draws energy back into your physical system. (This is ideal if you're air dominant.)
2. **Downward massage.** Place the heels of your hands over your closed eyes, fingertips at your hairline. Breathe. Then slide your palms down your face, neck, and torso. Make this a mini self-massage as you visualize drawing energy down your body. Press your thumbs into both hip creases and bend forward slightly. Rub your thighs, calves, and shins. To finish, press

your thumb into the sole of each foot. This is a beautiful way to celebrate yourself while physically massaging energy down through your body. (This is ideal if you're fire dominant.)

3. **Yogic seal.** Make a fist with the right hand. Cup the right fist in the left hand. Place the fist in the lower abdomen, an inch below the navel. Fold forward over your cupped hands with a straight spine. This seals energy into your belly. (This is ideal if you're earth dominant.)

To come out of meditation, dip your chin with your eyes still closed, as if gazing down. Then slowly open your eyes. Take in the color of the mat or floor, then slowly gaze around the rest of your room. If you still feel spacey, take a sip of water or lie down for a few moments.

Try each regrounding technique to see which one feels potent for you. Just one of these techniques may be enough to reground you. Or, if you tend to get light-headed or sense you have high air (*vata*), use two or three of these in combination. Your regrounding should be proportional to your meditation. After a long meditation, take a longer time to fully reground your awareness within your physical system.

After your regrounding technique(s), reconnect with the earthly world with one more deep belly breath. Now you can move forward in your day with calm, compassion, and purpose.

––––––––

When you first start meditating, you might feel stuck in step 1 and the first stages of step 2. You witness your mind and visualize the ball of light, but aren't yet connecting to anything bigger. That's OK! This can happen to the most experienced meditators. No one can *always* channel insights on demand. Observing your thoughts, practicing nonjudgment, and honing the skill of visualization has value on its own. Don't worry that you're "doing it wrong"—even if you don't sense anything mystical happening yet. Surrender. Remember "Let it go" (*ishvara pranidhana*)? Focus on the process. Not the outcome. Trust that as you keep practicing, a connection with this sense of universal calm and consciousness will form. Most things of value take time to master—it is a meditation *practice*. Not a meditation *perfect*. Give yourself grace. Be patient. Trust that you're doing it right.

You can practice meditation for three minutes or thirty. No matter what, the core components are the same: practice bearing witness to yourself, connect to the divine within, and then reground with renewed purpose and peace in your daily life. If you have only three minutes to practice, just do step 1. It counts even if you're not wearing yoga pants or sitting cross-legged. Just as with the breath (chapter 4), you can integrate principles from your meditation practice into your daily life from moment to moment: in a difficult conversation, between emails, or sitting in the car at a stoplight. Take a conscious, meditative pause between tasks.

YOGA HABIT: *Mini Meditation (Ten to Thirty Seconds)*

This meditation combines the breath awareness from chapter 4 with step 1 of our meditation framework: witnessing your thoughts. You can do these things together, in an instant, anytime. For example:

- In a heated conversation: Pause, breathe, and witness the binary lizard-brain response forming in your head *before* you say it.

- When you're at your laptop in a moment of overwhelm: Pause to label and categorize your thoughts (page 200) for one minute before continuing your tasks. Practice a full, complete breath.

- Waiting in a long line, stuck in traffic, sitting at the doctor's office: Exit your body and pretend you're the observer of your life from afar. Visualize watching yourself and your inner dialogue from the nearest tree, cloud, or rooftop.

PERSONALIZE YOUR MEDITATION

Once you're comfortable with these three foundational steps (*witness, connect, reground*), it's time to personalize your meditation practice. By adding a specific visualization or sound to the end of the ball of light visualization in step 2, you can adjust your meditation to invoke calm, clarity, or compassion—each of which will pacify a different dominant element.

Each of these variations summons a different energy. As always, feel free to experiment, and adjust based on what fits your mood in a given moment.

Prefer a guided audio for each meditation option? Download guided meditations at brettlarkin.com/practices.

For Calm (Ideal If You're Air Dominant)

- After completing the ball of light visualization, keep your eyes closed and picture a red triangle pointing down at your navel.

- Hold your focus on this shape (*yantra*).
- Ideal hand position: palms facedown on the thighs.

The triangle pointing toward the floor serves to anchor your energy and reground you. Red is the color associated with the earth element in yoga. This visualization is the ideal antidote for anxiety.

For Compassion (Ideal If You're Fire Dominant)

- After the first portion of the ball of light visualization, instead of holding the light in the center of the brain, bring it to your heart space.
- As you breathe in, silently think the mantra *hum*, but this time, feel the light at the center of your heart expand in all directions (forward and back, both sides, and up and down).
- As you breathe out, think *sa*. Coax this light gently back into your heart center.
- Over the course of ten to twelve breaths, expand this light around you. Visualize this glow from your heart radiating out, like a golden orb, then contracting back into your body. The light expands, then contracts. Match this pulsation of light— in and out—with the cadence of your breath.
- Optional: On days when you have more time to meditate, allow this light to expand like a sunrise, radiating bigger, brighter, and farther in every direction. Now the glow encompasses your whole room, apartment, town, everywhere. Everything and everyone is basking in the warmth and glow of this divine light.
- Ideal hand position: palms cupped and faceup in your lap, right hand under left.

For Clarity (Ideal If You're Earth Dominant)

- During the ball of light visualization, when you're envisioning the expansion of the ball of light in the brain center, use your index finger to gently tap the space between and above your eyebrows. This is your third eye center. Optionally, use your tongue to moisten your index finger before you tap. Tap two or three times to gain an awareness of this space, then set your hand back down.

- Gather your attention to focus on your third eye for several breaths.

- Feel a pinpoint of energy radiating there. This may feel like heat, white-gold light, or moisture; whatever you feel is fine.

- Focus all your energy on this single point while keeping your forehead wide and relaxed.

- If the analytical thinking mind comes online, chant the mantra *mung** to silence those thoughts and stay connected to universal intelligence.

- Release the mantra and reground when you're ready.

- Ideal hand position: palms faceup on the thighs, index finger and thumb touching.

The third eye center corresponds to the location of the pituitary gland in your brain, deep behind the spot you tapped. The pituitary

---

*This ancient mantra has no specific meaning. It's meant to sound like a gong reverberating inside your brain. *MUUUUUUUN-G!* Visualize a mallet hitting a golden gong in the center of your head. It should feel as if you're radiating purifying bright light from the center of the brain in all directions.

gland, the master gland of the body, secretes hormones that regulate your body's essential systems, resulting in your mood and how you feel right now.[4] The ancient yogis called this area the seat of our intuition, the point at which polarities dissolve.

Can't meditate for whatever reason? You can, as always, take each of these personalization techniques on the go. When you're out walking around, visualize a large upside-down red triangle at your navel (grounds excess air) or mentally think *MUUUUUUUN-G!* (soothes high earth and promotes clarity). Or imagine light radiating from your heart (ideal for high fire).

ASSEMBLE YOUR RITUAL

Drumroll moment! It's time to complete your worksheet!

Find a comfortable seat and practice the three steps of meditation (*witness, connect, reground*) for as long as time allows. To personalize, circle on your worksheet which flavor of the ball of light visualization worked best for you—the one for calm, clarity, or compassion.

FAQ

What if I keep falling asleep in Corpse Pose (Savasana) and never make it to meditation?

It means you need the rest. Thank your body for giving you what you needed in that moment. Strive to get more sleep and know that once you do, meditation will be easier. If you're *always* sleepy, talk to your health-care provider.

What if I get pins and needles in my legs?

Know that this is normal, especially when you're starting out. The best prevention is to sit up on a cushion and ensure your hips are higher than your knees. If numbness hits your leg or foot while you're meditating, keep drawing your focus inward. Gently straighten the leg that's bothering you, wiggle your toes, or change positions. You can always come into Corpse Pose for a few breaths and then return to your meditative seat once the sensation has passed.

How can I find time to meditate with my busy schedule?

If you have three minutes to scroll through your phone, you have three minutes to meditate. Just close your eyes, wherever you are, and observe your thoughts. Connect with your breath. Once you start feeling the benefits, you'll crave it.

What if I get a headache?

Pause the meditation, practice the regrounding techniques from step 3, and then take Corpse Pose. If you still have a headache, take a break and give yourself time to rest. Return to meditation and try a different technique the next time. Drink lots of water.

What are your thoughts on music?

I love music to accompany my personal yoga ritual, especially soothing nature sounds for Corpse Pose. But when it comes time to meditate, I find that music, or even background sounds like ocean waves, distracts me from the task at hand. My advice: Allow this to be the one moment in your day where you are input-free. Saturate yourself in silence even and perhaps *especially* if this is hard.

What if my family is loud, I get interrupted, or there's a really annoying noise?

Meditation is about practice, not perfection. Children may wander by, the washing machine may whir, jackhammers may start pounding outside your window. You may feel these noises are attracted to meditation! Observe your reaction to all these things by continuing to watch your thoughts. Notice what happens when your "annoyance program" flares up. Meditation gives you the gift of *noticing* your reaction. This is even more valuable when you're irritated. Remember, you're not meditating to *escape life*. You're meditating to gain an elevated awareness of how you *react to life*. Even monks had to deal with chirping birds.

What if I see [a white light/shapes/faces/insert your vision here]? What does it mean?

You may experience visual images while meditating, and this is no reason for alarm. Usually it means you've transcended the intellectual mind and are entering an even deeper state of meditation. This is a good thing. A white light or golden hue is common. If anything you see freaks you out, take a full, complete breath, do a regrounding technique, and open your eyes. Also, don't feel you're doing anything wrong if you don't "see" anything—ever. You may be more auditory and hear a particular sound or insight. Meditation affects each of us differently, but it uplifts us all.

IF YOU DO ONLY ONE THING

Build the muscle of witnessing your thoughts and growing your awareness. The physical practice of yoga exists to get you to this psychic destination—a place where you're able to pause and examine your habitual programming *without judgment*. In a word: meditation.

Know in your heart that the same spark of genius that created the birds, the trees, and the glorious sky is pulsating within you... waiting to forge a deeper relationship. Meditation is not about escaping. It's about embracing the greater intelligence *you have within you*. This is the divine you—calm, purposeful, and happy.

Meditation is so powerful that even if your practice is a hodge-podge throughout your week, you'll feel the start of a transformation. If you practice just bits and pieces of the techniques presented here, you cannot stay stuck. You'll uncover solutions and gain insights and compassion. You'll feel happier in seemingly magical ways.

CHAPTER 9

Your Life Is a Yoga Studio

Adapt When You're Strapped

Congratulations! You've handcrafted your very own twenty-minute personalized yoga ritual. You know how to observe your breath, transition into your winning warm-up, cultivate the opposite in your unique flow, go inward as you stretch, and, finally, meditate to channel the wisdom within you. But what happens when you don't have time for your ideal routine? Or when the seasons change and you notice that your energy shifts? Or you just broke your foot? Or you've been at it awhile and feel inspired to integrate new poses and shake things up?

Good news: The genius of the personal ritual you've created is that it's *modular*—meaning you can do it all together, in one progressive sequence, or reconfigure based on what's going on in your life. You can do certain sections as stand-alones or abbreviated rituals. Imagine your own yogic nesting Russian dolls—maybe you do all the pieces together, or maybe you just focus on one for today. Each individual segment by itself is a tool in your yoga tool kit.

Of course, the ideal is to flow through your whole ritual, from SIT to MEDITATE, every day. But I want to empower you to pick and choose segments of your ritual to eliminate, expand, or enhance based on what's going on in your life. Use this decision-making framework to adapt your ritual to the mood and moment you're in.

ADAPT YOUR RITUAL TO YOUR LIFE

We talked earlier about how every day is like an equation: Sleep + Food + Stress + Commitments + Family + Work + Physical Pain + Time + The State of the World = Your Available Energy. Your energy will vary throughout each day of your life. To stay consistent in your yoga practice, you need the tools to adapt. Deciding what segments of your sequence to skip or expand is surprisingly easy. Use these five guiding questions to adjust your ritual from day to day.

1. How did I sleep?

- If you're low on sleep, cut out the MOVE section, which is the most physically demanding. Stay close to the ground, prioritizing STRETCH and Corpse Pose instead.
- If you're well rested, expand your ritual, if possible (more on this in a minute)!

2. What's my stress level?

- If you're anxious or overwhelmed, prioritize SIT, WARM UP, or STRETCH and treat yourself to Corpse Pose (page 209) for as long as possible. These segments keep your body close to the ground and are especially soothing for your nervous system.
- If you're already calm, cool, and collected, challenge yourself by expanding and enhancing your MOVE and MEDITATE segments.

3. Am I in physical pain?

- If you're recovering from an injury, head to page 247 in the Yoga Adaptations Guide for specific suggestions on how to adapt your ritual.
- If you have a headache or cramps or feel a cold coming on, skip everything except your SIT or STRETCH segment and do Corpse Pose.

4. How much time do I have?

- Low on time? Do only your WARM UP segment, followed by either Corpse Pose or a brief MEDITATION.
- If you have the luxury of extra time, repeat your MOVE section, flowing through the same postures multiple times. Add in the ab work section at the end of MOVE. Luxuriate in your STRETCH poses for longer. Indulge in a ten-minute Corpse Pose.

5. What's my dominant element?

- If you're air dominant, prioritize SIT and STRETCH and take Corpse Pose. These sections work to ground your excess air by keeping you close to the ground. You'll be pulled to prioritize MOVE, but remember, the antidote you need is *stillness*.
- If you're fire dominant, prioritize your STRETCH and MED-ITATE segments and leave plenty of time for Corpse Pose, even though you'll want to cut these out first when you're short on time. These segments prioritize introspection and help you slow down. Expand them when you can.
- If you're earth dominant, WARM UP and MOVE are your top priorities. Your goal in a time crunch is to prioritize movement and flow. Always close with a brief Corpse Pose or a few moments seated and practice full, complete breaths.

The best part about your personal routine is that you can expand or contract the duration based on how long you have to practice. Elongate or cut sections based on your energy each day. Start by setting a timer on your phone for however many minutes you have to practice (for me, sometimes this is seven minutes). Next, take a deep breath and check in with yourself using the five questions above to guide you.

When in Doubt, Fall Back on These Three Simple Guidelines

1. The only segment of your ritual that cannot be performed in isolation is MOVE. Always WARM UP before you MOVE.

2. The segments SIT, WARM UP, STRETCH, and MEDITATE, as well as Corpse Pose, are all practices in their own right. You can perform any of them individually as the sum total of your practice, depending on your mood and energy level.

3. If all else fails, SIT. Focus on your breath first to notice how you're feeling. Ask yourself, *How do I feel? What do I want?* Remind yourself that your yoga practice is here to nourish you.

After you've been doing this awhile, dig a layer deeper if you can. Ask, *How do I feel? What do I want?* (*svadhyaya*) and *What's coming up next in my day? Would cultivating more air, fire, or earth help me best prepare?* See what comes up. Make the appropriate decision from there. Imagine you're an ER nurse who just finished an all-night shift on her feet. Likely you'd prefer to start with SIT. Imagine you've been trapped at a desk all day—you're desperate to start moving and don't have a lot of time. You'd immediately start flowing with WARM UP and perhaps SIT before meditation at the very end. Imagine you have high nerves, like Katie from chapter 6, and need to go onstage in two hours. You'd want to SIT and STRETCH in order to ground.

When life gets in the way and you don't have enough time to do your whole routine, instead of skipping—or feeling the overwhelm of starting from scratch—deconstruct what you already have. What modules match the moment you're in? You can devise your own totally unique abbreviated practice. Your completed worksheet is your cohesive ritual—your full-course meal. But feel empowered to create a modularized practice, using your worksheet like an à la carte menu, even if you order just a snack.

Let's look at a concrete example. Stacy, a fiery *pitta*, would complete her worksheet like this:

Uplifted Yoga® Personal Practice Worksheet

Stacy's Personal Yoga Ritual

Sit (*breath awareness*): Armpit breathing

Warm Up (*gentle movement*): Sufi Grind, Cat/Cow

Move (*heating and strengthening*): Hips and Inner Thighs Flow

Stretch (*winning wind-down*): Yin-Style Seated Forward Bend

Meditate (*The best part—relaxation*): For calm. For clarity. For compassion.

FAVORITE YOGA HABITS

- Do Less
- Park and Breathe
- Relinquish Control

She's chosen breathwork and postures that serve to slow her down, balance her naturally fiery tendencies, and help her practice self-compassion.

In her ideal world, Stacy would move through the full five-segment practice as her daily personal ritual. But this week Stacy has a huge deadline, and today she woke up late and anxious. She knows she needs to center herself stat. Like a short-order cook, she mixes up a recipe with only the grounding segments of her ritual. Her abbreviated routine is condensed to fifteen minutes and creates a soothing start to what was looking to be a rough day.

Mini Ritual to Calm Down

1. **Sit:** Armpit breathing (two minutes)
2. **Warm Up:** Cat/Cow (three minutes)
3. **Stretch:** Yin-Style Seated Forward Bend (seven minutes)
4. **Take Corpse Pose** (three minutes)

To create this mini ritual, Stacy cut out the MOVE and MEDITATE segments, which felt too energizing and mentally challenging. Instead of *skipping* her practice, she leveraged this abbreviated ritual to set herself up for success. Sometimes, though, Stacy doesn't even have fifteen minutes. In that case, she might create one of these quickie calming "yoga tonics":

• Just the SIT segment. She doesn't do anything else. Instead, Stacy does only her favorite calming breathing technique, for example, armpit breathing, taco breath, or a full, complete breath. She could pick one and do it in the car before turning on the engine. (Two minutes.)

- Only WARM UP. A quick Cat/Cow and Sufi Grind before she brushes her teeth is all there's time for. (Three minutes.)
- Doing a STRETCH. Sometimes the Yin-Style Seated Forward Bend is the ultimate one-pose calming practice. (Seven minutes.)

Do you see how, by picking and choosing pieces of what she learned, Stacy can create what's perfect for her in the moment? Do you see how you can do this too? Your ritual is flexible and easy to mold into whatever you need, day by day. You never have to skip your yoga practice. You just *adapt*.

Let's look at an opposite example. Stacy has a big day ahead: she's traveling for work and heading straight into meetings. She needs extra energy but doesn't want the caffeine crash that inevitably follows espresso shots. Instead, she whips up this yoga recipe:

Mini Ritual to Energize

1. **Warm Up:** Cat/Cow (two minutes)
2. **Move:** Hips and Inner Thighs Flow (five minutes)
3. **Add Ab Work** (one minute)
4. **Stretch:** Yin-Style Seated Forward Bend (seven minutes)

That's fifteen minutes of movement that will energize her with flowing standing poses, lunges, and abdominal work but cool and ground her at the end with the long-held forward fold. Even shorter energizing mini rituals might look like these:

- Only WARM UP and perform the ab work. That is enough to get your energy flowing. (Five minutes.)

- Only WARM UP and MOVE. Your heart will be pumping. (Eight minutes.)
- Only have a few seconds? Sit and do breath of fire. (One minute.)

Sometimes you'll want to have a meditation-only day. Maybe you're injured, tired, or feeling bloated on your cycle, and the last thing you want to do is yoga. *Remember the golden rule: Never avoid your practice, always adapt.* Here's what Stacy could practice on a day she feels the flu coming on:

Minimal-Movement Day

1. **Warm Up:** Cat/Cow (two minutes)
2. **Sit:** Armpit breathing (two minutes)
3. **Meditate:** For compassion (eight minutes)

That's a twelve-minute healing yoga infusion. Here are other minimal-movement or no-movement practices that take even less time:

- Just SIT: Do breathing only, focusing on your full, complete breaths. (Four minutes.)
- Just SIT and MEDITATE. Spend a few minutes with the armpit breathing, then do the meditation for compassion. (Ten minutes.)
- Just do Corpse Pose. Set a timer and rest. (Five minutes.)

EXPAND AND ENHANCE YOUR RITUAL

The house is clean and a babysitter just took your children to the park. You're miraculously faced with two empty hours. Rub your palms together with glee. Now is the time to practice an extended version of your personalized yoga ritual that fills your self-care gas tank to the brim. Here's how to transform your twenty-minute practice into a sixty-minute luxury class:

1. Repeat your MOVE section for a total of two to three times. This repetition gets you out of your head and into your body. Close your eyes as you flow through this section on your breath, multiple times.

2. Add the ab work on page 159 after your MOVE segment to strengthen your core.

3. Increase the time spent in your Yin-Style Seated Forward Bend to eleven minutes or more, and perform it after additional poses from your STRETCH segment.

4. Expand the time you spend doing breathwork by adding in a breathing technique before you meditate (see chapter 5). The more pranayama you can do before meditating, the easier and more profound your meditation experience will be.

5. Extend your Corpse Pose to ten minutes or even fifteen! Grab an eye pillow. Yes, you need this.

WHEN IT ALL FALLS APART

Look, even though you're equipped with an armload of yoga tools, there will still be days in which yoga poses and habits don't happen. This is completely normal. Remember: Nobody is committed all the time. Not even me! How much you *recommit* is what matters. When things go awry:

1. **Forgive yourself.** Immediately. Remind yourself that you're a human (not a robot) and that you're doing your best in an increasingly complex world.

2. **Don't obsess over the fact that you skipped a day.** Where your attention goes, your energy flows. So when you bemoan (internally or to other people) that you skipped your yoga practice, you're inadvertently giving that narrative momentum. One day off the mat becomes two days, three days, seven days, and then a month. Stay positive and look only forward (not back!). Ask: *How am I getting on my mat next?*

3. **Tell someone about your plan to practice yoga.** It's easy to break promises to ourselves. It's harder to fib to other people. Tell your friend, kid, or dog, "I'm getting on my yoga mat before dinner." This creates positive momentum (and subtle peer pressure). If nothing else, chant to yourself: "It's how much I *recommit* that matters."

Falling off the yoga wagon is normal. The action of showing up for yourself again is what builds confidence. Over time, an effortless yoga practice feels as ingrained as brushing (or flossing!) your teeth. Protect your yoga time—it's essential to show up as your best self. You are worth the effort! If you don't want to do this for *you*, do it for those around you. Don't rob the world of your most radiant, happy self by skipping the yoga that serves to balance you.

LEVERAGE YOUR YOGA HABITS

And of course, for all those moments when the very thought of meditating or stretching or doing one more Downdog sounds like your own personal version of hell, we have our Yoga Habits. Yep! It's OK not to make it to the mat all the time, or for life to get in the way. Yoga Habits are part of your yoga tool kit for a reason: These techniques empower you to turn challenging daily moments into something sensual, beautiful, and revitalizing. Leverage the Yoga Habits in this book to supplement, substitute for, or supercharge your physical practice.

Ever the go-getting, fiery *pitta*, I like to play a game in which I challenge myself to see how many off-the-mat Yoga Habits I can fit into each twenty-four-hour period. My record so far is twenty. The weirdest? Picture me on the bathroom floor, doing Cat/Cow with some hip circles for some In-Between Yoga (page 134) while my husband and I discuss travel plans as he shaves. Plus, I know I can reliably count on at least two toddler meltdowns a day to give me the opportunity to practice, and model, my magic breath ratio and the habit of relinquishing control. (No, we will not be arriving to the birthday party remotely on time.)

See if you can find ways to use your favorite Yoga Habits each day. Or maybe you want to start with mastering one and then layer in more. Whatever's going on, there's a habit in your yoga tool kit to support you.

UPLIFTED YOGA HABITS

YOGA HABIT	EXAMPLE
NOURISH YOURSELF (page 37)	After turning off your car's ignition, you pause and check in with yourself. You ask, *How do I feel? What do I need? What do I want?* before rushing to your next task.
CHOOSE TRANSFOR-MATION (page 40)	You're always late to appointments, so challenge yourself to arrive fifteen minutes early.
RELINQUISH CONTROL (page 47)	Your kitchen and living room look like they've survived a tsunami, but rather than trying to force everyone to fix it (or clean it up yourself), you let it go and head straight to bed.
BREATH AWARENESS (page 85)	Before falling asleep, you place a pillow on your belly and breathe deeply so it moves up and down.

MAGIC RATIO BREATH (page 94)	Decompressing after a conflict with your spouse, you inhale for five, pause, then exhale for five, pause.
SIGH IT OUT (page 97)	You feel aggravated writing a complex email, and, like a cartoon character, you extend your exhalation, sighing three times to calm down.
PARK AND BREATHE (page 113)	To help yourself transition from work to home, you practice taco breath for two minutes in your garage before going inside.
IN-BETWEEN YOGA (page 134)	You Cat/Cow before making dinner instead of mindlessly scrolling social media.
CULTIVATE THE OPPO-SITE (page 142)	You're craving a Snickers bar, but you make a spinach smoothie instead.
LAZY YOGA (page 184)	You watch your favorite TV show while doing Ankle to Knee.
DO LESS (page 188)	It's 5:30 p.m., and even though there's more work to be done, you walk away from your computer.
LET IT GO (page 194)	Someone frustrates you, and you shake it off by going for a walk around the block instead of phoning a friend to complain.
MINI MEDITATION (page 217)	In the bathtub you sit back and close your eyes to practice the ball of light visualization.

Do you see how on any average day you can practice Yoga Habits, incorporating more serenity into your life from moment to moment? Even if you never set foot on a yoga mat? Alone, each of these habits may seem inconsequential. However, over the course of days and weeks, you'll be surprised at how different you feel. All these small actions add up to bring calm and compassion into your life and the lives of people around you.

WHAT TIME OF DAY SHOULD I PRACTICE?

Short answer: Whenever you want! Adapt your yoga ritual to your schedule. Practice anytime you can. That said, it's easier to build a habit when you do something at the same time each day. Consistency in the time you choose to practice your ritual helps ensure that it happens. That could be in the morning after you brush your teeth, after dinner when the plates are clean, or before you eat lunch. Ancient yogis used to say the period just before the sun rose (4:00 or 5:00 a.m.) was the most potent time to practice yoga. But I've had my most earth-shattering practices in the middle of the afternoon! Find what's doable for you.

Waking up before my family and doing my twenty-minute ritual plus ten minutes of meditation works best for me. But this wouldn't work for someone who works the night shift. Strive to create any consistent ritual time that works for your personal life, then "yoga snack" on abbreviated rituals and Yoga Habits throughout the day. Get creative. Remember, you can do yoga in the morning if you're pressed for time and practice meditation on its own before bed. In especially stressful periods of my life, I've meditated for five minutes three times a day (morning, noon, and night) in addition to doing my morning yoga practice. The goal is to stop thinking of yoga as one thing that needs to take tons of time. Sprinkle joyful yoga glitter throughout your whole day, and see how it draws your happiest self forward.

And voilà! We did it! You're the proud creator and owner of your very own yoga tool kit. Now that you've assembled a yoga ritual that's personal to you, please feel empowered to disassemble it, tweak it, and reassemble it to cater to your current mood and moment. Your practice is meant to evolve with you, not stay the same. Don't forget that you can always head over to the Yoga Adaptations Guide on page 241 for more specific guidance and suggested flows for beginners, those dealing with acute injury, people who are pregnant or breastfeeding, and more.

LIVE YOUR BEST LIFE

Equipped with your yoga tool kit, you now have the skills to unearth the loving BFF within you. The friend who wants to truly *listen* to how you are feeling (*svadhyaya*) and asks, "How are you feeling? What do you need? And what do you really want?" The friend who tells you, "This is not your fault and not your problem. Let go. Breathe. Relinquish control!" (*ishvara pranidhana*). The friend who holds you accountable and challenges you with, "Don't fall into that same old trap. Grow! Cultivate something new and different" (*tapas*).

All the yoga poses, all your personalized segments in their limitless combinations, lead to this inner knowing—this best friend inside you—your calmest, happiest self. You're now empowered with dozens of tools to channel your purpose and your joy. Like an archer, reach into your yoga quiver and find the particular arrow that slays the challenge you're facing today. Each time you do, you'll gain more intimacy with your expansive, dazzling, yogic self. Over time you can access this joyful identity—the real you—even in your lowest, nonyoga moments. Your unique personal practice guides you toward inner clarity, confidence, and compassion—ultimately, a happier and fulfilled you!

Little things really do add up. The results of your practice are cumulative. Listen to your body. Be your own instructor and work with the adaptations that make the most sense for YOU. Note how you feel after each practice. All this serves to inform how you'll adjust your routine. Honor your direct experience—this is what creates the magic in yoga. Keep adapting, experimenting, and adjusting your flows so they become uniquely YOU. Not you yesterday. But you right now, in this exact moment. Yoga is not a linear journey from beginner to advanced. It's a continuous cycle inward, with peaks, valleys, recommitments, and higher peaks. Trust yourself and trust the process.

Immersed in yoga your way, you now relinquish control of what you can't control anyway and commit to the most enduring and important relationship—the one with yourself. You were born to be a gift to the world and to those around you. Not by striving and controlling, but by honoring a commitment to show up as your most radiant, balanced self. Practicing your yoga, your way, is that commitment.

I used to wake up each morning afraid of the future, especially during my rock-bottom year. Cloaked in anxiety before I even lifted my comforter, I'd begin brainstorming ways to mitigate potential disasters. This sense of overwhelming dread seeped into my intimate relationships, draining the pleasure and suffocating the intimacy. To be honest, I'm still struggling with anxiety, worry, and fear—but unlike before, I now have an abundance of yogic tools that I can whip out on the mat, off the mat, no matter where I am or how long I have. No emotion, no part of me, is too big for these tools. The old way I used to practice yoga, trusting someone else to tell me what to do, stopped serving me. So I reinvented what yoga meant to me, flipped the script on how and where it could be practiced—and it's changed my entire life.

These days, when fear and anxiety creep in, I remind myself I am powerful and well-equipped: My yoga tool kit is waiting to be leveraged. I've harnessed a powerful set of yogic practices, rooted in ancient wisdom, proven throughout the ages, that modern science endorses more each day. This immediately makes me feel less alone. And that's what I want for you too. These tools unite us. Your yoga tool kit empowers you to meet yourself where you are. Even if the moment is ugly. Go *live* your yoga. Get creative with your ritual. Manifest your happiest, best self every day. The beauty of a personalized yoga ritual is the positive ripple effect that flows throughout your whole life. Eventually, you barely notice; it's part of who you are now—your transformed self: Calm. Purposeful. Happy.

Stay in Touch!

Enjoyed this book? I would love to welcome you into my upcoming online yoga teacher trainings, Yoga for Self-Mastery program, and Uplifted Yoga membership and connect with you on social media @larkinyogatv. I hope to bliss out with you on yoga, in real time, very soon!

Visit brettlarkin.com.

Yoga Adaptations Guide

The only constant in life? Change. Major life events—starting yoga for the first time, dealing with an acute injury, getting pregnant—all require you to further adapt your personal practice. In this section you'll find additional tips and specific adaptation recommendations to help you reshape and restyle your ritual.

ANXIETY, STRESS, AND OVERWHELM

Anxiety and stress signal you have too much fire (*pitta*) or air (*vata*), even if it's not your dominant *dosha*. This is common, since our fast-paced society promotes these elements. The good news? Multiple studies have proven that yoga reduces stress and anxiety.[1] The quickest way to rebalance is to ground your body by getting more limbs in contact with the ground. Here are my top tips for those of you struggling with anxiety, stress, and overwhelm.

Tips

- **Take your yoga tool kit outside.** Anytime you can practice your Yoga Habits or personal ritual outside, it's a double win. Take a full, complete breath while walking around your neighborhood, in the woods, or standing barefoot in a patch of grass. Practice your SIT segment in your backyard, a park, or under a tree. Meditate in the sun. Move your whole mat outside if you have a patio, deck, or other flat space on which to practice. Connecting and reintegrating with nature has been proven to relax your nervous system.[2]
- **Take yoga breaks.** Pause intentionally throughout the day and lie down for Corpse Pose, even just for five minutes. Use the Yoga Habits Sigh It Out, Do Less, Relinquish Control, and Mini Meditation multiple times a day.
- **Be gentle with yourself.** This is not the time to mix new poses into your sequence. Instead, elongate your STRETCH section or practice it in isolation. Identify and indulge in poses that soothe and nurture you.

- **Turn off the lights.** Keeping the room dim as you practice will make your yoga feel extra nourishing and more like a refuge. For any poses where you're lying on your back on the ground, place a weighted pillow over your eyes.
- **Breathe breathe breathe.** Remember, the breath is the internal "thermostat" controlling your mood. Use the "system override" of your breath to wipe out overwhelm by working with the magic ratio (page 92) in your full, complete breath and in taco breath. Three-part breath and armpit breath are also excellent techniques you can practice anywhere (literally!) to calm down.

Adaptations

- Prioritize soothing breathwork and poses in which your body is close to the floor. Cut out everything that isn't supportive to grounding. Favor these antianxiety poses and techniques in your personal sequence, or perform them in isolation:
    - Cat/Cow (*Chakravakasana*)
    - Warm Up and Grounding Flow or Calming Flow
    - Yin-Style Seated Forward Bend (*Paschimottanasana*)
    - Ball of light visualization for calm
    - Reground
- **Prioritize Corpse Pose.** Elongate when possible. This pose is extremely grounding and the ultimate way to give your body, mind, and spirit the deep rest it needs during your moments of stress, anxiety, and overwhelm.
- Avoid:
    - Breath of fire (*kapalbhati*)
    - Energizing Flow
    - Abdominal work

MENSTRUATION

During menstruation the energy in your body moves downward as the uterine lining is shed. During this time you want to work *with* the body's natural intelligence rather than against it. This means you want to avoid poses and breathing techniques that move your energy upward. In Ayurveda, menstruation is a time to orient your attention inward and practice extreme self-care. As tempting as it may be, don't skip your practice. Doing yoga on your cycle has been proven to *ease* menstrual symptoms.[3] Instead, *adapt*. Here are my tips to adjust your personal ritual when you're on your cycle.

Tips

- **Move slowly.** Prioritize ease. You're more sensitive and intuitive on the first three days of your cycle. Don't push yourself into action. Think of menstruation as your ultimate opportunity to go inward and practice self-awareness. It's a self-imposed time-out from regular life that's built into your physical body. Now is the time to soak up the rest and relaxation you deserve. Remember: You're a person, not a robot. Your period is a physical signal to slow down, take a break, and recharge. You have the rest of the month to go-go-go if you choose.

- **Always make it to your mat.** Even if all you can manage is Corpse Pose with a hot-water bottle on your belly, challenge yourself to rest on your yoga mat instead of your bed. Spending time on your physical yoga mat, even if you're not doing a physical yoga practice, honors your commitment to yourself and your dedication to the self-awareness that leads to self-care (*svadhyaya*). It's also a beautiful moment to meditate on "let it go" (*ishvara pranidhana*)—the idea of surrender and relinquishing control. As the body sheds its uterine lining and a new monthly cycle begins, ask yourself, *What else can I release?*

- **Embrace change.** No two women are exactly alike. Even within your own body, no two periods are exactly the same. Tune in to your body and your energy. Trust your intuition. Find movements and mini rituals that feel good for you. Depending on your energy, you might want to just do your WARM UP and STRETCH sections, or just SIT. Gentle movements close to the ground can ease premenstrual cramps and low-back pain. The length of a woman's period is highly variable, and how long you'll want to adjust your practice is also very personal. Many women overhaul their rituals to be restorative (the WARM UP or STRETCH section only) on the first three days of their cycle, then slowly transition back to their full personal practice on the last two days of their cycle. Others may prefer to adapt their practice for eight days or longer. Adapt your ritual in the days leading up to your period, inviting in slower, gentler movements. You know your body best. You're the designer. Everything is up to you.

Adaptations

- Your period is a great time to practice the three-part breath (page 101), which releases physical tension and can even ease low-back pain when practiced with a bolster under the knees, lying down on the floor.
- Avoid breath of fire during menstruation. It moves your energy up, which is the opposite of your natural flow (more details on page 111).
- Skip or modify your MOVE segment, which builds heat and raises your energy, if you feel fatigue. Make your time on the mat all about receiving nourishment from your practice. More *being*, less doing.

- Poses that help lessen symptoms like cramps, low-back pain, and headaches, either during your period or before, include:
  - Cat/Cow (*Chakravakasana*)
  - Sufi Grind
  - Spinal Flex
  - Baby Cobra (*Bhujangasana*)
  - Head to Knee Forward Bend (*Janu Sirsasana*)
  - Seated Twist (*Ardha Matsyendrasana*)
  - Butterfly Stretch (*Baddha Konasana*)

Did you know? You can use Ayurveda's *doshas* to better understand your menstrual cycle. An air (*vata*) period is a lighter flow or an irregular cycle. A fire (*pitta*) period is fast, furious, and shorter in length. An earth (*kapha*) period is heavier and lengthier. Although this time is ultimately about turning inward (not cultivating the opposite), it's good to be aware of your flow type and what that might mean for your overall well-being. If you have a fiery *pitta* period, do you need to slow down in life in general? Or if you have an airy *vata* period, how can you get more grounded throughout the entirety of your cycle?

INJURY RECOVERY

Do you know the number one reason people flock to yoga? Low-back pain! From a yogic perspective, your injury is a self-development opportunity. Reframe it as an occasion to cultivate new skills and to grow as a person. Remember those karmic moments (page 12) that force us to grow? Your injury is here to teach you something.

I often hear from my Uplifted members that they're injured and so they can't practice yoga. While it's true that their injuries may prevent them from practicing various physical components of yoga, as we all know, yoga is way more than just poses! Please allow me to remind you: If you're breathing, you can do yoga. You have thirteen Yoga Habits at your disposal, as well as breathwork and meditation, which require no movement. Injury recovery is a great time to tune in to the more subtle aspects of your yoga practice. Focus on deep breathwork and meditation, the powerful tools that normally get shortchanged. If you're dealing with an injury that prevents you from practicing your personal ritual the way you would like, here are my ideas for you:

Note: Make sure to consult your physician and care team as you incorporate yoga into your healing process.

Tips

- **Props, props, and more props.** Don't push your body if it's injured. After one of my yoga teacher training instructors broke her foot outside of class, she became incredibly creative with her props. She discovered all sorts of new ways she loved to move on the floor. Support your body during your practice with as many props as possible and see what emerges.
- **Be a body detective.** Once your doctor has cleared you to do yoga, get curious. See how your body feels. Your body may tell you what it needs in your recovery process. Beyond your symptoms, what habitual bracing patterns on the mat or in life could have resulted in this injury? Are your shoulders always up at your ears? Do you hold tension in your neck or jaw? Dig deeper to identify the root cause.
- **Consider bodywork.** Visit a myofascial release therapist and explore alternate healing forms. Acupuncture or physical therapy may help you find the root cause of your injury and a more direct route to recovery.

- **Take ownership of your healing journey.** Many people can feel like victims to their diagnoses. However, your yoga mat is an area where you remain empowered and in charge. The rectangle of your mat is a space where you can tap into your identity as a healer. Use the Yoga of Awareness to make the most of this karmic moment. Can you reframe it? Perhaps your seemingly random injury is here to evolve your personality in some way. Maybe you need to overcome excess fire (*pitta*) and your injury is here to help you learn how to finally slow down. Perhaps you need to learn to receive and let others care for you. Perhaps you need to learn how to relinquish control in a deeper way. Or overcome your aversion to stillness. According to yogic philosophy, your injury is here to aid you in mastering a skill that leads you forward to your highest self.

Adaptations

- The fundamental rule of injury management is if it hurts, *don't do it*. Take a nurturing, gentle approach with your yoga practice. If your breath becomes constricted, back off. Remember, you are the prime mover in your healing. The yoga mat is a place where YOU are in charge. This can bring comfort in a world of doctors and diagnoses where you may feel out of control and disempowered. On the yoga mat, you're the author of your healing story. Focus on what you *can* do.
- Focus on the SIT and MEDITATION segments of your ritual. When you're trapped in bed or on the couch, this may be your best opportunity to take your breathwork and meditation practice to the next level. Breathwork doesn't promote only mental health, but physical health too. Remember my hunky Croatian crush? The one who sparked my interest in yoga?

He had the body of an Olympian god and he practiced only breathwork. A strong diaphragm positively affects *all* your muscles and organs. You may not be moving in poses, but your yoga practice still can accelerate your recovery.

- Skip your MOVE segment if needed. Do only seated poses (if you're able to).
- Create a no-arms version of your practice. This means eliminating Downdog, Cat/Cow, Planks, and Baby Cobra and focusing on standing poses like Goddess Pose, Triangle Pose, Pyramid Pose, Tree Pose, and Warrior 2.

Injury-Specific Adaptations

- Spinal injury: Poses like Ankle to Knee, Baby Cobra, and Seated Twist both strengthen and release tension in the spine.
- Shoulder injury: Cat/Cow and Dog-to-Plank Flow will strengthen your shoulder muscles once you've been cleared to practice.
- Wrist injury: Prioritize pressing your knuckles into the mat to create space in the wrist joint. Use a YogaJelly or a folded mat under your wrist for support (see page 262). Are there ways to use your forearms instead of your hands in a pose?
- Knee injury: Avoid putting pressure on the knees, or pad the knees in poses on all fours. Engage the muscles along the backs of your legs and around the knee to create more space and stability in your knee joint. Bend your knee slightly in poses that ask for a straight leg, hugging your thigh muscles in toward the bone.
- Chronic illness: Practice the Yin-Style Seated Forward Bend daily—it deeply relaxes the nervous system. Use the ball of light visualization meditation to visualize healing energy moving up and down your spine.

WEIGHT LOSS

Many people come to yoga for weight loss and toning. I want to remind you that you do not need to be any size or shape to do yoga or to reach your highest self. However, if weight loss and toning are goals for you, yoga can support that journey.

It seems counterintuitive, but restorative yoga, akin to the poses in your STRETCH segment, has been proven to aid in weight loss *more* than heating, sweaty flows.[4] These postures soothe your nervous system, reducing cortisol, the stress hormone that increases abdominal fat. When it comes to keeping your body healthy, a regulated nervous system is the key. You can achieve this through relaxation. Many students looking to lose weight ask me if yoga counts as cardio exercise. My short answer is, technically, no. But due to yoga's nervous system benefits, it may be just as beneficial.[5] If you happen to be doing cardio exercise as part of a weight-loss regimen, yoga provides much-needed stretching and cross-training. Here are my top tips and adaptations for adjusting your personal practice for a toning and weight-loss goal.

Tips

- **Practice in the morning.** The new science of chrononutrition (adapting your diet to your biological clock) explains that, just as eating a nutritious higher-calorie breakfast helps support your overall health,[6] doing your ritual every morning at the same time makes the practice you're already doing more effective for weight loss by syncing it with your circadian rhythm.

- **Anytime you're hungry but want to fast, get on your mat and move.** Poses with flowy movements like Cat/Cow and Sufi Grind help distract you from hunger pains if you're fasting or resisting a snack. Anytime you feel a craving coming on and it's not time to eat, jump on your mat and move your body instead. If you're truly hungry, of course, always eat.

- **Practice more than once a day.** Do your complete personal ritual in the morning. Add breath of fire or abdominal work in the late afternoon. Practice deep restorative poses and meditation before bed.

- **Make full, complete breathing a priority.** Sending your diaphragm down on an inhalation and drawing it up on an exhalation doesn't only strengthen your back and core muscles. It also stimulates your digestion. According to the University of Michigan, diaphragmatic breathing helps you rest and digest, alleviating issues like abdominal pain, constipation, and bloating.[7] This keeps your gastrointestinal tract healthy and your process of elimination strong! You can't breathe your way to your weight-loss goal, but it can tremendously support your body.

Adaptations

- Do lots of breath of fire (two to five minutes multiple times a day) to detoxify your system and enhance your digestion.

- Repeat your MOVE flow for a total of two to five times to increase your heart rate and burn more calories in your practice.

- Add in abdominal work at the end of your MOVE segment. This builds heat in the body and cultivates a strong core.

- Soothe your nervous system with Corpse Pose (*Savasana*) and the Yin-Style Seated Forward Bend, either at the end of your ritual or later, before bed.

- Bigger bodies: Widen your stance (left to right on your mat) in all standing postures so the feet are wider than the hips. You can even widen your stance in Downdog.

BEGINNERS

Brand new to yoga? Most beginners want to follow along with videos they find online since they have no idea how to start practicing at home and want to be talked through what to do. The problem? Usually the instructor moves too fast and the poses are too complex. You disconnect from your breath and go into mental overload trying to keep up. This leads to frustration, or, worst of all, injury, which is not at all what we're aiming for.

You're light-years ahead since you've already designed your own personalized practice from scratch. This empowers you to deeply tune in to your body and move on your own breath cadence from day one. No longer are you trapped, following along with classes that aren't right for you (as most students do *for years*). To help you discover a sustainable practice you can commit to for the long term, here are my top tips if you're new to yoga.

Tips

- **Less is more.** When in doubt, pick simpler poses for your worksheet. At this stage, don't worry about challenging yourself too much physically. You want to focus on your breath. If there's anything you take away from this book, I want it to be this: *breath over poses!*

- **Repetition is your friend.** Adding too many tools too soon to your personal practice forces your intellectual mind to the forefront, divorcing you from your deepest breath and a more meditative state. Instead, choose simple postures and stick with them until you achieve mastery. This allows you to develop a relationship with your *most* important muscle—the diaphragm.

- **Leverage props.** Use yoga blocks, blankets, cushions, and pillows to help you achieve the Uplifted Yoga Golden Rule: *Length in the spine.* Oh! And repeat after me: "I don't need fancy props to get started." Household items work just as well. If you don't have a yoga strap, use a belt or scarf. Don't have a cushion? Grab a throw pillow. Props are not training wheels you grow out of. The most experienced yogis use them throughout their journeys. You don't need to invest in expensive equipment.

- **Use a mirror.** Your ultimate goal is to look inward. But to check your form in any pose, as an intermediate step, practice alongside a mirror. Notice if your spine is long (or not) and grab a prop or adjust your body accordingly. I urge all my online yoga teacher training students to work with a full-length mirror. It's the best way to learn how each pose looks in *your* body. Over time you'll be able to feel when you have found your perfect alignment, without any visual aids.

- **Don't compare.** Delete from your brain the images you've seen of yoga on Instagram, on TV, or in magazines. That's someone else's practice, not *yours*. It doesn't matter if your heels don't reach the ground in Downdog. Who cares if your arm doesn't touch the floor in Side Angle Pose? Don't judge yourself. Your yoga is for *you*, not for public display. Focus on the sensations in your body and connect with your deepest breath. Dim the lights or close your eyes once you know your sequence. A calming ambience can help you tune inward.

- **Set the goal of practicing for thirty days in a row.** Neuroscience tells us it takes thirty days for a habit to form. I promise, if you commit to doing your personalized practice for thirty days in a row, you will see (and feel) your progress. Tell everyone around you that you're doing this. Let them hold you accountable! After thirty days, you'll never want to go back to your nonyoga life.

Adaptations

- In your SIT, WARM UP, and STRETCH segments, sit on a cushion if you're not used to sitting on the floor. You want your hips above your knees so you can achieve length in your low back.

- In all-fours poses, like Cat/Cow, pad under your knees with a folded blanket or towel. Extra padding makes everything feel easier on your joints.

- During your MOVE segment, take an extrawide stance on your mat (left to right) for poses like Aura Painting, Lizard, and Pyramid. Placing your feet wider than your hips helps you gain stability while performing these movements. You can also better support yourself in poses like Goddess and Tree if you lean against a wall or doorframe for support. Every part of your home is here to support your practice.

- Always work with blocks in these standing poses, even if you think you don't need them:

  ○ **Triangle Pose:** Place a block standing vertically so it's as high as possible in front of your shin and press your hand into it to find a longer spine.

  ○ **Side Angle Pose:** Use a block under the bottom hand to find more length in the spine.

  ○ **Wide-Leg Forward Fold:** If folding forward all the way makes you light-headed, place your hands on blocks, a chair, or a coffee table. Then fold just halfway down so your spine is parallel to the floor (rather than bending all the way down).

- Performing Downdog with length in the spine takes a lot of upper-body strength! Glance at your Downdog in front of a mirror to ensure your spine isn't rounding and think, *Booty toward the ceiling, knees deeply bent, torso toward thighs* as you find your long spine.

- Simply holding Dog for three to five breaths at a time (don't even enter Plank Pose) may be enough for your first thirty days.

If and when you decide to rock forward into Plank, you can bend your knees once you're there (so your knees just hover off the ground). At the same time, draw your abs actively up and in. This might feel a LOT better on your low back than Plank Pose with straight legs.

- Bigger body or problems with balance? Take the feet wider apart and/or practice near a wall for extra support.

PREGNANCY

A common misconception is that pregnant women must modify their yoga practice because they're "weak," when actually, pregnant women are superheroes (secretly building a brand-new life within them while still juggling all their usual commitments) and highly intuitive. Common pregnancy symptoms, like food cravings, food aversions, extreme fatigue, and morning sickness, are actually a result of your body's increased awareness and hypersensitivity. In my Pregnant & Powerful Prenatal Yoga Program, I describe how the pituitary gland, the master gland ancient yogis associated with intuition, physically *enlarges* during pregnancy.[8] When you're carrying a child, you're literally more intuitive than you've ever been before. So there's never been a better time to trust yourself and follow your cravings!

From an Ayurvedic perspective, pregnancy is a state of excess fire (*pitta*), even though it may not feel like that in early pregnancy. Getting out of bed can be a struggle! In yoga philosophy, the element of fire resides within the navel. When you're pregnant, especially in trimesters two and three, you're literally exploding outward from that area. As you create life within you, you're radiantly powerful and on fire, literally—*pregnant women run hot*!

Obviously, as your baby grows and your body changes, your yoga practice will need to adapt. But let's be clear: If you skip or adapt anything, it is not because you're "weakened"; it's because you need to cultivate the opposite of the fiery energy of creation glowing inside you. Lean into your yoga practice when you're expecting. Studies have found that yoga eases stress, anxiety, and depression during pregnancy, while also reducing pain and discomfort.[9] Here are my top tips for adjusting your personal practice while pregnant:

Tips

- **Focus on stability, not flexibility.** During pregnancy, a hormone called relaxin loosens the ligaments (especially around your pelvis) to create more space for your baby's adorable head to work its way through the birth canal. Your ligaments stretch as your body prepares to give birth, so, while pregnant, you may find you can bend into certain poses deeper than ever before. Please, DO NOT do that! You risk overstretching, which could result in tendon tears or permanent ligament damage. Instead, cultivate the opposite and prioritize strength and stability. This will keep your body balanced and strong, help you avoid injuries, and soothe common pregnancy discomforts like low-back pain and round ligament pain in the hips or groin.

- **Allow yourself to eat, drink, rest, and stay cool throughout your practice.** Drink lots of water and take breaks as needed. Don't push yourself (or judge yourself!). Position yourself in the coolest part of the room if you run hot.

- **Don't compare.** Every woman is unique, and each of her individual pregnancies is also unique. Don't compare this experience to how other women are experiencing pregnancy, or even to your own prior pregnancies. Strive to personalize your ritual with a focus on how you're feeling in *this* moment, in *this* pregnancy. Adjust as much as needed so you can make it to your mat each day.

- **Connect with your baby.** Allow your yoga ritual to become an intimate bonding time for you and this blessed new soul. Place one or both hands on your belly in poses like Triangle, Side Angle, Goddess, and Warrior 2. Send your breath down toward your baby (even if she's kicking you!).
- **Practice self-awareness.** You're doing yoga with a completely different body—one that changes dramatically each trimester. Don't expect anything to feel the same as before. Midway through your second trimester, you may want to completely change your personal practice. Start a brand-new worksheet, take the quizzes in this book again, and redesign your ritual for who you are *now*.
- **Amp up your breath.** In the third trimester, it can sometimes feel as if your diaphragm and your baby are competing for space, resulting in a shortness of breath. Recommit to breathing as deeply as possible, even if your diaphragm has a smaller range of motion than before. Remember, each time you take a full, complete breath, your baby receives more oxygen too.[10] What a gift for both of you! The slower and more deeply you breathe, the more your nervous system shifts into a state of calm. Your baby feels that sense of safety; your body is its home! Become a ninja at full, complete breathing. Throughout your yoga practice, as you inhale, think about sending your breath down to "cocoon" your baby. Ensure your diaphragm is moving down as you inhale and up as you exhale.

  Beyond nurturing your unborn child, your ability to breathe deeply will prove invaluable during labor. Birth is an experience of getting comfortable with discomfort. It's wildly unpredictable. Your number one tool for controlling the uncontrollable is your breath. Now is a great time to start—or elongate—your breathwork and meditation practice. As I found in my own two labors, your ability to leverage your breath will help you feel confident and strong.

Adaptations

- Be mindful as you transition from sitting to standing. Changes in blood volume cause many women to feel light-headed. With your new pregnant body, your proprioception (your perception of how your body is moving through space) may be off. Avoid sudden movements, especially up and down. Take extra care as you transition between yoga poses, especially in getting up from and down to the floor. Instead of standing or sitting in one big motion, break it into two or three smaller chunks. For example:
  - **From Sitting to Standing:** From sitting, come onto all fours. Press into a wide-legged Downdog. Slowly walk your hands toward your feet. Bend your knees generously and place your hands or elbows on your thighs. Take several breaths in this flat-back position before slowly pressing your hands into your thighs to come fully upright.
  - **From Standing to Sitting:** Reverse the steps above, walking your hands down your legs and bending your knees to sit, using your hands for support. Alternatively, stand with your back to the wall and slide down the wall to transition to seated.
- During pregnancy, your hips slightly widen and your sense of balance changes. Take a wider stance (left to right on your mat) in all standing postures so your feet are *wider* than your hips. You can even widen your stance in Downdog.
- Lean against a wall for poses like Triangle, Warrior 2, Goddess, and Side Angle and for transitioning from standing to sitting, especially in your third trimester. Lean against the wall or hold the back of a chair to help yourself balance in Tree Pose.

- Include an extralong Corpse Pose (fifteen minutes whenever possible). During the first trimester, it's OK to lie on your back during Corpse Pose. In the second and third trimesters, take Corpse Pose lying on your left side with a cushion between your knees and a blanket or bolster under your head. This position ensures optimal blood flow for you and your baby.
- Poses and breathing techniques to **include:**
  - Full, complete breaths
  - Taco breathing (*sitali/sitkari*)
  - Cat/Cow (*Chakravakasana*; also a great position to labor in!)
  - Sufi Grind
  - Butterfly Stretch (*Baddha Konasana*)
  - Head to Knee Forward Bend (*Janu Sirsasana*)
  - Corpse Pose (*Savasana*; on the left side starting in the second trimester)
- Poses and breathing techniques to **avoid:**
  - Breath of fire (*kapalbhati*)
  - Darth Vader breath (*ujjayi*)
  - Three-part breath (*krama*)
  - Boat Pose (*Navasana*)
  - Aura Painting
  - Baby Cobra (*Bhujangasana*)
  - Seated Twist (*Ardha Matsyendrasana*)

MENOPAUSE AND HEALTHY AGING

Menopause is a time of profound transition, and many women find it can be the most empowering stage of their lives. While this stage of transformation brings physical change, it's also a time of reawakening, shedding old identities, and embracing new ones. You may discover a new sense of independence and the courage to boldly step into your own power.

A study by researchers at the *American Journal of Obstetrics & Gynecology* in 2014 found that menopausal women who did a daily twenty-minute home yoga practice reported fewer hot flashes, improved sex, and a better quality of life.[11] Aren't you glad you have your personalized practice ready to go?

Many women report that menopause disrupts their sleep and daily schedule. To counterbalance this, prioritize structure and routine in your daily life—from what time you go to sleep to what you choose to eat to when you make time to practice each day. Eliminate as many variables as you can. Now is a great time to prioritize doing your full yoga ritual, from start to finish, every day at the same time. It will be your rock—a constant—as your body goes through major hormonal changes.

Bone degeneration is also a common concern during this period. While it's part of the natural aging process, studies have shown that just twelve minutes of yoga every day improves bone mineral density in older adults with osteoporosis, reducing the risk of falls and fractures.[12] Your yoga also serves to enhance your posture, balance, coordination, and range of motion.

Tips

- **Hug muscle to bone.** It's especially important to activate your muscles in each and every yoga pose. Since you're going through a major life change, it's time to focus on stability. Strength, basic mobility, and balance should be your focus. The best way to incorporate these is through more standing poses (your MOVE section).

- **Add in more balancing postures.** The best way to prevent falls is to train for balance. Beyond Tree Pose (page 156), you might choose to adapt all-fours postures into a balancing act. For example, after Cat/Cow, lift one arm off the ground, one leg off the ground, or your opposite arm and leg together! Balancing poses strengthen your core and the small stabilizing muscles in your feet and ankles. For standing balances, have a chair or wall nearby for extra support.

- **Realize that what feels good may have changed.** As your body transitions to a new phase, so will your practice. Experiment with props, even if you've never used them before. Keep a pillow, bolster, or blanket nearby. Always place your knees or booty on something cushy. Ease up if you feel any discomfort. Don't push yourself. Be open to experimentation and adjust your personal practice accordingly.
- **Breathe through hot flashes.** Taco breath is the ideal go-to breath technique for menopausal women. Practice it often to cool down and calm down.

Adaptations

- For arthritis, carpal tunnel, or wrist pain, practice Cat/Cow and all-fours postures with your hands in fists rather than with your palms flat on the mat. Skip Downdog and Plank, or elevate your wrists higher than your fingers to eliminate discomfort. You can do this by folding over the top of your mat so the heels of your hands are on the mat and your fingers are on the floor. Some people also choose to purchase YogaJellies (round jelly pads to use under wrists, knees, and hips for softness) to elevate wrists higher than fingers.
- Poses and breathing techniques to prioritize:
  - Taco breathing (*sitali/sitkari*)
  - Armpit breathing (*padadhirasana*)
  - Cat/Cow (*Chakravakasana*)
  - Spinal Flex
  - Warrior 2 (*Virabhadrasana 2*)

- Tree Pose (*Vrikshasana*)
- Baby Cobra (*Bhujangasana*)
- Abdominal work
- Seated Twist (*Ardha Matsyendrasana*)
- Corpse Pose (*Savasana*)

Ready for More?

If all of this leaves you craving more, I've got you covered. Join my Uplifted membership community for monthly teachings and to get instant access to hundreds of hours of customized instruction from yours truly.

Visit brettlarkin.com.

Yoga Poses, Breathwork, Meditations, and Habits

SIT (*Breath Awareness*)

Taco breathing or *sitali/sitkari*—calming

Darth Vader breath or *ujjayi*—focusing

Three-part breath or *krama*—rejuvenating

Alternate-nostril breath or *nadi shodhana*—clarifying

Armpit breath or *padadhirasana*—healing

Breath of fire or *kapalbhati*—energizing

WARM UP (*Gentle Movement*)

Cat/Cow (*Chakravakasana*)

Spinal Flex

Sufi Grind

Sun Breath

Dog-to-Plank Flow

MOVE (*Heating and Strengthening*)

Low-Back Saver Flow/Grounding Flow (Vata*)*

- Baby Cobra (*Bhujangasana*)
- Child's Pose (*Balasana*)
- Pyramid Pose (*Parsvottanasana*)

- Tree Pose (*Vrikshasana*)
- Warrior 2 (*Virabhadrasana 2*)
- Wide-Leg Forward Fold (*Prasarita Padottanasana*)

*Hips and Inner Thighs Flow/Calming Flow (*Pitta*)*

- Aura Painting
- Lizard Pose with Clamshell Arms
- Moving Goddess Pose
- Triangle Pose with Arm Circles (*Trikonasana*)
- Wide-Leg Forward Fold (*Prasarita Padottanasana*)

*Backbend Flow/Energizing Flow (*Kapha*)*

- Moving Baby Cobra (*Bhujangasana*)
- Aura Painting
- Side Angle to Reverse Warrior (*Parsvakonasana* Flow)
- Tree Pose with Arms Up (*Vrikshasana*)
- Dynamic Bridge (*Setu Bandha Sarvangasana*)

Bonus: Abdominal Work to Add Heat

- Static Forearm Plank Hold
- Boat Pose (*Navasana*)

STRETCH (*Winning Wind-Down*)

- Head to Knee Forward Bend (*Janu Sirsasana*)
- Butterfly Stretch (*Baddha Konasana*)
- Ankle to Knee—Reclined Pigeon
- Seated Twist (*Ardha Matsyendrasana*)
- Yin-Style Seated Forward Bend (*Paschimottanasana*)—Three Minutes Minimum

MEDITATE

Sit: On a Chair, on a Cushion, in Hero's Pose (Virasana*)*

- Ball of light visualization
- For calm (ideal if you're air dominant)
- For compassion (ideal if you're fire dominant)
- For clarity (ideal if you're earth dominant)

Reground

- Palm rubbing
- Downward massage
- Yogic seal

YOGA HABITS

- Nourish Yourself (page 37)
- Choose Transformation (page 40)
- Relinquish Control (page 47)
- Breath Awareness (page 85)
- Magic Ratio Breath (page 94)
- Sigh It Out (page 97)
- Park and Breathe (page 113)
- In-Between Yoga (page 134)
- Cultivate the Opposite (page 142)
- Lazy Yoga (page 184)
- Do Less (page 188)
- Let It Go (page 194)
- Mini Meditation (page 217)

Glossary

akhara: Forerunner to the modern yoga studio created by Krishnamacharya, the father of modern yoga.

alignment: "Perfect" alignment in yoga doesn't exist, since each body is unique. Instead, the primary goal is to get you into your intuitive healing zone. In Uplifted Yoga, essential alignment starts with a full, complete breath rather than with mastering *more* poses. In the poses, the goals are to prioritize length in your spine and link your breath to movement.

asana: The physical practice of yoga—movement of the body, postures.

Ashtanga: A type of yoga created by Pattabhi Jois based on what he studied with Krishnamacharya: a physically rigorous series of postures with the breath cadence counted out loud.

Atman: Your unique spirit; Universal Consciousness, but with your individuality—your unique identity—attached.

Ayurveda: A traditional holistic system of medicine that originated in India more than three thousand years ago and is focused on balance in the body. Sanskrit for "life knowledge."

Bikram Yoga: A style of yoga, with a strict sequence of poses performed in a room heated to a very high temperature, created by Bikram Choudhury.

Brahman: Universal Consciousness; the yet-to-be-thought-of wisdom residing in cosmic intelligence. The raw data of the universe where polarity dissolves. Deep, limitless love.

dosha: Ayurveda explains how each of us is uniquely made up of three elements called the *doshas*—fire, earth, and air—with one element being dominant.

full, complete breath: The full, complete breath is the optimal anatomical way to breathe. The magic ratio of five-and-a-half-second inhalations and five-and-a-half-second exhalations is the optimal rhythm in which to perform it. This is the anatomically correct way you were born to breathe (before society and trauma retrained you into shallow-breathing stress patterns).

hatha: Often translated from Sanskrit as "discipline of force"—a style of yoga focused on mastery of the body, practiced slowly, with focus on the breath, controlled movements, and stretching.

ishvara pranidhana: Surrender. Relinquishing control. Diverting all the energy you expend attempting to control people or outcomes. Instead, the energy is channeled into the benevolent faith that everything will work out. Choosing your faith over your fear.

kapalbhati **aka breath of fire:** Energizing, heating, and detoxifying. This rapid-fire breathing technique increases the level of oxygen in your system—making it especially good for earthy *kaphas*.

karma: The process of unwinding and dissolving the habitual stress responses and fear-based programs we picked up or inherited in this lifetime.

karmic moment: A moment when you use the Yoga of Awareness to choose something other than your habitual response. A moment when the universe provides you with an opportunity to make a choice from your highest self instead of your habitual patterns.

krama **aka three-part breath:** A deep inhalation with three pauses as you fill up with breath; this helps retrain your diaphragm toward anatomical efficiency.

Tirumalai Krishnamacharya: Renowned as the father of modern yoga (1888–1989); repositioned yoga from a solely spiritual practice for priest boys and ascetics to a physical practice available to the masses.

kriya-yogah: Described in sutra 2.1, yoga in action happens when you practice *svadhyaya* (self-awareness), *tapas* (transformation), and *ishvara pranidhana* (surrender), both on and off the mat.

kundalini: "Coiled energy"—a yoga style that includes chanting, singing, breathing exercises, and repetitive poses for the purpose of activating kundalini energy at the base of your spine.

magic ratio breath: Breath that consists of inhaling for five and a half seconds and exhaling for five and a half seconds.

meditation: Willingness to witness all the thoughts in your mind without judgment.

nadi shodhana **aka alternate-nostril breathing:** An energy-harmonizing exercise: breathing through the right and left nostrils alternately. A balancing pattern for all three elements.

padadhirasana **aka armpit breathing:** Breathing that balances the nervous system like alternate-nostril breathing but doesn't require touching the face or alternating nostrils.

personal practice: A ritual that soothes your unique mind, body, and spirit, pacifying your dominant element—designed to balance your energy and help you uncover your highest self. Often also called *sadhana*, which translates to "daily spiritual practice."

prakriti: The "balanced" you that you were meant to be before fear and insecurity crept in. You achieve it again when the elements within you return to however they were balanced when you were born. Returning to this unique mix of elements, your "balance birthright," liberates the authentic you—the unfettered, passionate, magnetic childhood version of you, brimming with grace, purpose, and joy.

pranayama: Breath control—the profound yogic science of changing how you feel through specific breathing patterns. Using the breath to override or change the way you're thinking.

props: Blocks, straps, bolsters, blankets, or other household items to be used during the physical practice of yoga so you feel nourished and supported.

regrounding: Channeling energetic wisdom from yoga and meditation back down into your daily life. The goal in regrounding is to siphon the universal wisdom down through your physical body so you can act on it as you move through this world.

restorative yoga: A practice in which the poses are held in stillness for much longer than in other styles of yoga. Your body is fully supported by props here.

Savasana: Corpse Pose—a posture of total relaxation, lying on one's back; the essential resting pose in yoga.

sitali/sitkari **aka taco breathing**: An open-mouthed inhalation that is cooling and calming (making it ideal for those with fire, *pitta*, as their dominant *dosha*). Use this breath anytime you're overheating, angry, or just in need of some chill.

sutra: Translated from Sanskrit as "string" or "thread." Bite-size nuggets of yogic wisdom reduced by Patanjali to the fewest possible words.

svadhyaya: Self-awareness that leads you to look within and discover the best way to nourish and honor yourself in the present moment.

tapas: The uncomfortable actions you take that go against the grain of your negative habitual tendencies. *Tapas* evolves you as a person and transforms your life for the better.

ujjayi **aka Darth Vader breath**: Sanskrit for "one who is victorious"; this technique generates heat and focus, making it ideal for our earthy *kaphas*. Use this breath anytime you need to hone your focus, stay calm, and solve problems.

Uplifted Yoga: A yoga-in-action style developed by Brett Larkin that prioritizes variety, personalization, and adaptability, giving you the self-awareness to adapt your practice to the moment you're in—physically, mentally, emotionally, or spiritually. You can practice Uplifted Yoga even if you never set foot on your mat.

vinyasa: Translated from Sanskrit as "to place in a specific way"—a yoga style that focuses on linking your inhalations and exhalations to how you're moving your

body through a continuous flow of movement, often at one breath per movement cycle.

vrakriti: How you're operating right now, subconsciously bound by learned patterns from your family and stressful life circumstances that create a restrictive
shell. This shell prevents you from embodying the authentic and highest self
you're here to reclaim.

yin: A yoga style that holds seated yoga poses for extended periods of time in stillness to stretch your interconnective tissues. The long holds also provide space
to observe your emotions, thoughts, and physical sensations.

Yoga Habits: Yogic wisdom that you can sprinkle like glitter throughout your
whole day and that helps you cultivate *svadhyaya* and embody *tapas* and *ishvara
pranidhana* from moment to moment.

Yoga of Awareness: A practical yoga redefined by Brett Larkin that brings a new
energetic frequency to an event in order for you to find a creative way through;
the ability to widen the lens of your awareness to introduce more breadth,
depth, and creativity into how you're approaching your problems.

yoga tool kit: Personalized Yoga Habits, breathwork, poses, and segments that you
can use both on and off the mat, in any amount of time, to shift your energy.
Yogic techniques that restore you to balance—fast.

yogic adaptability: The self-awareness to adapt your practice to the moment
you're in—physically, mentally, emotionally, or spiritually.

Acknowledgments

Writing a book was the idea of my husband and my Uplifted Yoga team. Thank you all for your support, confidence, and encouragement. I never would have had the wherewithal or patience to undertake a project of this size without your cheerleading. Dr. Cindy Childress, thank you for your incredible help in shaping the proposal and finding my agent, Michele Martin. From our first conversation, I knew it had to be you, Michele, who helped bring this book into the world. Immense gratitude to my talented editor Hannah Robinson. Hannah, working with you has been almost too easy. We always seem to agree. Your feedback and suggestions have been invaluable. Thank you for advocating for this book and all the hours you've put into the process. Co-creating with you has been a dream.

Caitlin Sammons supported me in hundreds of ways throughout this project. From drafting chapters, organizing my lectures and notes, researching, proofreading, quiz-taking, and perfecting every aspect of the manuscript from concept through to completion. Caitlin, I love who you are as a person. Thank you for being my co-pilot on this project. My brilliant mother, Ellan Cates-Smith, the woman who taught me how to write, also spent countless hours (often at the expenses of playing with her own grandchildren!) fine-tuning every chapter. Mum, you have helped me so much with every aspect of this book. I am insanely grateful.

I've had the privilege of learning about yoga from so many incredible teachers and I want to acknowledge them here. Thank you, Sarah Platt-Finger, Alan Finger, Wendy Newton, Peter Ferko, Mona Anand, Douglass Stewart, Kristin Leal, and everyone who trained me and believed in me at ISHTA Yoga in New York City. Elena Brower was a pivotal teacher and mentor for me as I first gathered the confidence to teach and start my family. Jason Crandell, Kia Miller, and Guru Singh, thank you all for your wisdom and your light.

I feel blessed to be supported by a rock-star team of humans inside my Uplifted Yoga business. Thank you for caring about our students and our work in the world as much as I do. Stephanie, Sara, and Mhel, you have been my rocks and believed in me since day one. Jen, thank you for sharing a "yoga brain" with me. Kristi, Katrina, Kristin, Danni, and Erica, thank you for the depth of wisdom you bring to our online teacher trainings. Marquis, Talena, Andrea, Yadav, Louise, Jessy, Amanda, Kate, Barbie, all of you have supported and impacted me, the business, and our students. Thank you to my home team and everyone who helps with my kids: Marie, Elena, Sylvia, and Anna.

Lastly, thank you to my husband, who is always taking care of me, looking out for me, problem-solving for me, and delivering food to my office. You are the only man for me, forever. Thank you to my father, who instilled in me an entrepreneurial spirit. Dad, I feel your presence within me and around me all the time. You are here. And thank you to every single yoga-lover, Uplifted Member, Uplifted Yoga Teacher Training Graduate, and YouTube viewer who has practiced with me. If you have ever left a comment or review, or shared my classes, or participated in our programs, I am in your debt. You are "my people" and I feel so honored to be a part of your journey. Let's all keep spreading the light.

Notes

PART I

Chapter 1

1. Drake Baer, "One of America's Most Beloved Authors Just Told Us Her 'Number One Life Hack' for Lasting Relationships," *Business Insider*, August 26, 2015, https://www.businessinsider.com/brene-browns-biggest-life-hack-is-a-simple-phrase-2015-8.
2. Christian Keysers and Valeria Gazzola, "Hebbian Learning and Predictive Mirror Neurons for Actions, Sensations and Emotions," *Philosophical Transactions of the Royal Society of London,* Series B, Biological Sciences (April 28, 2014): 369 (1644), doi: 10.1098/rstb.2013.0175.
3. Mark Wolynn, *It Didn't Start with You: How Inherited Family Trauma Shapes Who We Are and How to End the Cycle* (New York: Penguin, 2016).
4. Gary Kraftsow, *Yoga for Wellness: Healing with the Timeless Teachings of Viniyoga* (New York: Penguin, 1999).
5. "Ayurveda," Health, Johns Hopkins Medicine, accessed July 8, 2022, https://www.hopkinsmedicine.org/health/wellness-and-prevention/ayurveda.
6. Ibid.
7. Ibid.
8. Swami Krishnananda, *The Path to Freedom: Mastering the Art of Total Perception*, https://www.swami-krishnananda.org/freedom.html.
9. Ibid.

Chapter 2

1. Subhamoy Das, "The Four Stages of Hinduism," Hinduism, Learn Religion, last updated August 10, 2018, https://www.learnreligions.com/stages-of-life-in-hinduism-1770068.

2. T. K. V. Desikachar, *The Heart of Yoga: Developing a Personal Practice* (Rochester, VT: Inner Traditions,1995).

3. Sri Swami Satchidananda, *The Yoga Sutras of Patanjali* (Integral Yoga, 1978).

4. Ibid.

5. Ibid.

6. Tasha Eurich, "What Self-Awareness Really Is (and How to Cultivate It)," *Harvard Business Review*, January 4, 2018, https://hbr.org/2018/01/what-self-awareness-really-is-and-how-to-cultivate-it.

7. Satchidananda, *Yoga Sutras of Patanjali.*

8. Jennifer Rioux, "A Complex, Nonlinear Dynamic Systems Perspective on Ayurveda and Ayurvedic Research," *Journal of Alternative and Complementary Medicine* 18, no. 7 (July 2012): 709–18, https://www.ncbi.nlm.nih.gov/pmc/articles/PMC3405450/.

9. "Balance Your Health Through Ayurveda," Ayurveda, The Art of Living, accessed September 18, 2022, https://www.artofliving.org/in-en/ayurveda/what-is-ayurveda/dosha-imbalance.

10. Satchidananda, *Yoga Sutras of Patanjali.*

11. Laura Doyle, *The Empowered Wife: Six Surprising Secrets for Attracting Your Husband's Time, Attention, and Affection* (Dallas, TX: BenBella Books, 2017).

Chapter 3

1. Desikachar, *The Heart of Yoga*, p. 79.

2. Kate Samuelson, "What to Know About Bikram Choudhury, the Yoga Guru with an Arrest Warrant," *Time*, May 26, 2017, https://time.com/4795788/yoga-guru-bikram-choudhury/.

3. Mark Singleton, *Yoga Body: The Origins of Modern Posture Practice* (New York: Oxford University Press, 2010).

4. Ann Pizer, "What Is Restorative Yoga?" Yoga, Verywell Fit, accessed July 8, 2022, https://www.verywellfit.com/what-is-restorative-yoga-3566876.

5. Nora Isaacs, "Is a Kundalini Awakening Safe?" *Yoga Journal*, May 4, 2021, https://www.yogajournal.com/yoga-101/types-of-yoga/kundalini/kundalini-awakening/.

6. "Explore the Ancient Roots of Yoga," Arts and Culture, Google, accessed July 8, 2022, https://artsandculture.google.com/story/explore-the-ancient-roots-of-yoga/rAKCRDl92CPuJg.

7. Wikipedia, s.v. "Asceticism, accessed July 8, 2022, https://en.wikipedia.org/wiki/Asceticism.

8. Singleton, *Yoga Body.*

9. Colin Hall, "Asana, Self-Mortification, and the Myth of the Hardworking Yogi," Yoga International, accessed July 8, 2022, https://yogainternational

.com/article/view/asana-self-mortification-and-the-myth-of-the-hardworking
-yogi.

10. *Britannica*, s.v. "Industrial Revolution," last modified October 27, 2022, https://www.britannica.com/event/Industrial-Revolution.

11. Conor "The History of Fitness," Physical Culture Study, published November 30, 2018, https://physicalculturestudy.com/2018/11/30/the-history-of-fitness/.

12. Lance C. Dalleck and Len Kravitz, "The History of Fitness," University of New Mexico, accessed July 8, 2022, https://www.unm.edu/~lkravitz/Arti cle%20folder/history.html.

13. James D. Lutz, "Lest We Forget, a Short History of Housing in the United States," American Council for an Energy-Efficient Economy, accessed July 8, 2022, https://www.aceee.org/files/proceedings/2004/data/papers/SS04_Panel1 _Paper17.pdf.

14. "The Electric Light System," National Park Service, last modified February 26, 2015, https://www.nps.gov/edis/learn/kidsyouth/the-electric-light-system -phonograph-motion-pictures.htm.

15. "Explore the Ancient Roots of Yoga," https://artsandculture.google.com/story /explore-the-ancient-roots-of-yoga/rAKCRDl92CPuJg.

16. Singleton, *Yoga Body*.

17. Ibid.

18. Ibid.

19. Ibid.

20. "the Mother of Martial Arts That Combines Massage Techinques [sic] and Ayurveda," Fitness, TheHealthSite.com, accessed July 8, 2022, https://www .thehealthsite.com/fitness/kalaripayattu-the-mother-of-martial-arts-that-com bines-yoga-and-ayurveda-218625/.

21. Wikipedia, s.v. "Mallakhamba," accessed July 8, 2022, https://en.wikipedia .org/wiki/Mallakhamba.

22. Svatmarama, *The Hatha Yoga Pradipika*, trans. Brian Dana Akers (Woodstock, NY: YogaVidya.com, 2002).

23. Singleton, *Yoga Body*.

24. Ibid.

25. Catherine S., "The Evolution of Group Fitness," *Be Well*, published March 23, 2017, https://www.bewellauburn.com/digest/2016/11/8/the-evolution-of -group-fitness.

26. Ibid.

27. Singleton, *Yoga Body*.

28. "The Gift of Rest—Eye Pillow Benefits for Stress and Sleep," YogaClicks, accessed July 8, 2022, https://yogaclicks.com/blogs/product-guides/the-gift-of-rest-eye -pillow-benefits-for-stress-and-sleep.

PART II

1. Gail Matthews, "Goals Research Summary," Dominican University of California, https://www.dominican.edu/sites/default/files/2020-02/gailmatthews-harvard-goals-researchsummary.pdf.

Chapter 4

1. Wikipedia, s.v. "Asana," accessed July 31, 2022, https://en.wikipedia.org/wiki/Asana.
2. Jaimie Epstein, "Physical Fitness Was Never the Purpose of Yoga," Yoga International, accessed July 31, 2022, https://yogainternational.com/article/view/physical-fitness-was-never-the-purpose-of-yoga.
3. James Nestor, *Deep: Freediving, Renegade Science, and What the Ocean Tells Us About Ourselves* (New York: Mariner Books, 2014).
4. "Stress System Malfunction Could Lead to Serious, Life Threatening Disease," Newsroom, Eunice Kennedy Shriver National Institute of Child Health and Human Development, published September 9, 2002, https://www.nichd.nih.gov/newsroom/releases/stress.
5. Sulagna Misra, "Learning Body Positivity from a 700-Year-Old Hindu Statue," *Racked*, December 10, 2015, https://www.racked.com/2015/12/10/9880964/body-positive-parvati-hindu-goddess-museum.
6. Hidetaka Hamasaki, "Effects of Diaphragmatic Breathing on Health: A Narrative Review." *Medicines* 7, no. 10 (October 15, 2020): 65, https://www.ncbi.nlm.nih.gov/pmc/articles/PMC7602530/.
7. Bruno Bordoni and Emiliano Zanier, "Anatomic Connections of the Diaphragm: Influence of Respiration on the Body System," *Journal of Multidisciplinary Healthcare* 6 (2013): 281–91, doi: 10.2147/JMDH.S45443.
8. "Stress System Malfunction https://www.nichd.nih.gov/newsroom/releases/stress.
9. Rachael Rifkin, "How Shallow Breathing Affects Your Whole Body," *Headspace*, accessed June 2, 2022, https://www.headspace.com/articles/shallow-breathing-whole-body.
10. Desikachar, *Heart of Yoga*.

Chapter 5

1. Daniel J. Levitin, "Why It's So Hard to Pay Attention, Explained by Science," *Fast Company*, September 23, 2015, https://www.fastcompany.com/3051417/why-its-so-hard-to-pay-attention-explained-by-science.
2. Desikachar, *Heart of Yoga*.
3. Ibid.

Chapter 6

1. Helen Hope, "A Bit (Too Much) of a Stretch: The Risks of Overstretching," *Dance Spirit*, October 17, 2019, https://dancespirit.com/risks-of-over stretching/.

2. Gaétan Chevalier, "Earthing: Health Implications of Reconnecting the Human Body to the Earth's Surface Electrons," *Journal of Environmental and Public Health* (January 12, 2012), doi: 10.1155/2012/291541.

3. Eleesha Lockett, "Grounding: Exploring Earthing Science and the Benefits Behind It," Healthline, last modified August 30, 2019, https://www.health line.com/health/grounding.

4. Jenny Savage, "Yoga Twists, the Ins and Outs," EkhartYoga, accessed June 2, 2022, https://www.ekhartyoga.com/articles/practice/yoga-twists-the-ins-and -outs.

Chapter 7

1. "Myofascial Release," Our Approach, Trauma Recovery Clinic, accessed July 31, 2022, https://traumarecoveryclinic.com/our-approach/myofascial -release/.

2. Hope, "A Bit (Too Much) of a Stretch."

3. Jacqueline Buchanan, "Top 5 Benefits of Forward Folds," DoYou, last modified October 4, 2015, https://www.doyou.com/top-5-benefits-of-forward-folds -90857/.

4. "Lose Weight with Restorative Yoga," *Yoga Journal*, October 23, 2013, https://www.yogajournal.com/poses/types/restorative-types-of-yoga/lose-weight-with -restorative-yoga/.

5. Eline S. van der Valk, Mesut Savas, and Elisabeth F. C. van Rossum, "Stress and Obesity: Are There More Susceptible Individuals?" *Current Obesity Reports* 7 (2018): 193–203, https://doi.org/10.1007/s13679-018-0306-y.

Chapter 8

1. C. S. Andreassen, "Online Social Network Site Addiction: A Comprehensive Review," *Current Addiction Reports* 2 (2015): 175–84, https://doi.org/10.1007 /s40429-015-0056-9.

2. Joseph Troncale, "Your Lizard Brain: The Limbic System and Brain Functioning," *Psychology Today*, April 22, 2014, https://www.psychologytoday.com/us /blog/where-addiction-meets-your-brain/201404/your-lizard-brain.

3. Tom Ireland, "What Does Mindfulness Meditation Do to Your Brain?" *Scientific American*, June 12, 2014, https://blogs.scientificamerican.com/guest-blog /what-does-mindfulness-meditation-do-to-your-brain/.

4. "Pituitary Gland," Health, Johns Hopkins Medicine, accessed June 2, 2022, https://www.hopkinsmedicine.org/health/conditions-and-diseases/the-pituitary -gland.

Yoga Adaptations Guide

1. Masoumeh Shohani et al., "The Effect of Yoga on Stress, Anxiety, and Depression in Women," *International Journal of Preventative Medicine* 9 (February 21, 2018), doi: 10.4103/ijpvm.IJPVM_242_16.

2. "11 Scientific Reasons Why Being in Nature is Relaxing," *Mental Floss*, October 12, 2015, https://www.mentalfloss.com/article/60632/11-scientific-reasons -why-being-nature-relaxing.

3. Jennifer Oates, "The Effect of Yoga on Menstrual Disorders: A Systematic Review." *Journal of Alternative and Complementary Medicine* 23, no. 6 (2017): 407–17, doi: 10.1089/acm.2016.0363.

4. Adam M. Bernstein et al., "Yoga in the Management of Overweight and Obesity," *American Journal of Lifestyle Medicine* 8, no. 1 (2014: 33–41, https://journals.sagepub.com/doi/abs/10.1177/1559827613492097.

5. Janice Neumann, "Yoga May Benefit Heart Health as Much as Aerobics," *Reuters*, December 26, 2014, https://www.reuters.com/article/us-health-yoga -cardio-trials/yoga-may-benefit-heart-health-as-much-as-aerobics-idUSKBN0 K40Y520141226.

6. "Chrononutrition: The Importance of Meal Timing," *Wellness Today: Integrative Nutrition,* Health & Wellness Blogs, Institute of Integrative Nutrition, last modified January 25, 2021, https://www.integrativenutrition.com/blog /chrononutrition-meal-timing.

7. "Diaphragmatic Breathing for GI Patients," Digestive and Liver Health, University of Michigan Health, https://www.uofmhealth.org/conditions-treatments /digestive-and-liver-health/diaphragmatic-breathing-gi-patients.

8. A. D. Elster, T. G. Sanders, F. S. Vines, and M. Y. Chen, "Size and Shape of the Pituitary Gland During Pregnancy and Post Partum: Measurement with MR Imaging," *Radiology* 181, no. 2 (November 1991): 531–35, https://pubs.rsna.org /doi/10.1148/radiology.181.2.1924800.

9. Marilyn Wei, "Yoga in Pregnancy: Many Poses Are Safer Than Once Thought," Harvard Health, Harvard Medical School, published December 29, 2015, https://www.health.harvard.edu/blog/yoga-in-pregnancy-many-poses-are -safer-than-once-thought-201512298898#.

10. Carrie Noriega, coauthor, "How to Increase Oxygen Flow During Pregnancy," Health, wikiHow, last modified July 22, 2022, https://www.wikihow.com /Increase-Oxygen-Flow-During-Pregnancy.

11. Susan D. Reed et al., "Menopausal Quality of Life: RCT of Yoga, Exercise, and Omega-3 Supplements," *American Journal of Obstetrics & Gynecology* (November 11, 2013), doi: 10.1016/j.ajog.2013.11.016.

12. Yi Hsueh Lu et al., "Twelve-Minute Daily Yoga Regimen Reverses Osteoporotic Bone Loss," *Topics in Geriatric Rehabilitation* 32, no. 2 (April/June 2016): 81–87, https://journals.lww.com/topicsingeriatricrehabilitation/fulltext/2016/04000/twelve_minute_daily_yoga_regimen_reverses.3.aspx.

About the Author

Brett Larkin attracts a devoted global following as a yoga teacher trainer, healer, and breakthrough entrepreneur. To help more people tap into the limitless power of yoga, Brett created the world's first yoga certification program online, running it live, interactive, and in real time. After launching her award-winning YouTube yoga channel and her Uplifted Online Yoga Teacher Trainings, within three years Brett was running a multimillion-dollar business. Brett's first career focused on human movement, where she created top-selling fitness and dance video games and worked with Beyoncé and her team to explore interactive dance fitness games for girls. Brett's yoga has been featured on NBC's TV news channel in Seattle, in podcasts, and in media outlets like *USA Today, Gaia, Well+Good, Greatist, Forbes*, Entrepreneur .com, and *POPSUGAR*. Join her nurturing online courses, communities, and certification programs at brettlarkin.com.